"This book is a gem – full of soli ....passionate approach to help women and providers understand the powerful connections between maternal mental health, eating disorders, and recovery from perfectionism and shame. In the introduction to her book, Dr. McCabe shares an inspired thought she had when she was coming out of her own postpartum crisis, as she realized that not only could she make it through this rite of passage, but also that she would recover and help other women. This book is a skilful and encouraging vehicle for that inspiration and her message: Hold on to the thread that Recovery is Possible. You are not alone. This book provides that help, adding an essential loving voice and practical tools for maternal mental health and recovery."

—*Wendy N. Davis, PhD, Executive Director of*
Postpartum Support International

"Using both her professional and personal lived experience, Dr. Linda Shanti deftly describes how eating disorder recovery and motherhood are profound initiations into whole new ways of being. With compassion and deep wisdom, she offers insight and guidance for those navigating the overlapping and simultaneous challenges of these transformative processes. I highly recommend this book to anyone seeking understanding and support on this journey!"

—*Anita Johnston, PhD, author of* Eating in the Light of the Moon

"It's about time we challenge the images of perfect bodies, perfect pregnancies, and perfect parenting and Recovery Mama *delivers*. For women struggling with body image or disordered eating, pregnancy is potentially transformative, either motivating recovery or fuelling a relapse. In this era of pregorexia, any woman navigating this new life stage will treasure Recovery Mama – it should be on every childbirth preparation resource list!"

—*Margo Maine, licensed psychologist, co-founder of the*
Maine & Weinstein Specialty Group, senior editor and author of
Eating Disorders: The Journal of Treatment and Prevention

of related interest

How to Kiss Goodbye to Ana
Using EFT in Recovery from Anorexia
Kim Marshall
ISBN 978 1 78592 464 4
eISBN 978 1 78450 841 8

I Can Beat Anorexia!
Finding the Motivation, Confidence and
Skills to Recover and Avoid Relapse
Dr Nicola Davies
ISBN 978 1 78592 187 2
eISBN 978 1 78450 459 5

Eating Disorder Recovery Handbook
A Practical Guide to Long-Term Recovery
Dr Nicola Davies and Emma Bacon
ISBN 978 1 78592 133 9
eISBN 978 1 78450 398 7

Maintaining Recovery from Eating Disorders
Avoiding Relapse and Recovering Life
Naomi Feigenbaum
ISBN 978 1 84905 815 5
eISBN 978 0 85700 250 1

Ed Says U Said
Eating Disorder Translator
June Alexander and Cate Sangster
ISBN 978 1 84905 331 0
eISBN 978 0 85700 677 6

The Recovery Mama Guide to

Your Eating Disorder Recovery *in* Pregnancy *and* Postpartum

—— ♡ ——

Linda Shanti McCabe

Foreword by Carolyn Costin

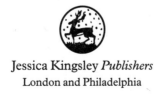

Jessica Kingsley *Publishers*
London and Philadelphia

First published in 2019
by Jessica Kingsley Publishers
73 Collier Street
London N1 9BE, UK
and
400 Market Street, Suite 400
Philadelphia, PA 19106, USA

www.jkp.com

Copyright © Linda Shanti McCabe 2019
Foreword copyright © Carolyn Costin 2019

Front cover image source: Linda Shanti McCabe.

Library of Congress Cataloging in Publication Data
A CIP catalog record for this book is available from the Library of Congress

British Library Cataloguing in Publication Data
A CIP catalogue record for this book is available from the British Library

ISBN 978 1 78592 829 1
eISBN 978 1 78592 590 0

Printed and bound in the United States

When a baby is born, so is a mother.
You need to grow her, along with your baby.

Contents

Foreword

——— ♡ ———

Author and clinician Linda Shanti McCabe has broken new ground in *The Recovery Mama Guide to Your Eating Disorder Recovery in Pregnancy and Postpartum*.

As someone who has recovered from an eating disorder and treated eating disorder clients for three decades, I'm so grateful for this book. I will tell my colleagues about it, add it to my eating disorder library, and recommend it to clients who have had or have an eating disorder, who become pregnant.

Linda takes her targeted audience through territory where two of the worlds they live in collide. Having lived in both worlds – having an eating disorder and having a child – Linda has successfully written about how to navigate the terrain when these two worlds collapse into one. Before now, good reading material that speaks to the challenges that arise in individuals with these particular circumstances has not been available.

From gaining weight, to body image, what and how much to eat, others' comments about weight, feeling out of control of one's body, changes in hormones, and much more, pregnancy brings many of the same issues that are faced in eating disorder recovery. Up until now there has been little written for pregnant individuals with a current or history of an eating disorder to turn to for help, understanding, and gentle wise advice. Not any more.

Linda gives wise council, stopping short of specific direct advice. The book is more about helping women she calls "recovery mamas" look wisely at the issues, feel empathized with, and learn what they can and cannot do to help themselves. For example, Linda points out that just as a person can plan out their own eating disorder recovery but cannot actually control it, so, too, it goes for pregnancy and birth. The book helps readers find the right balance between creating plans and letting go of them, while also getting needed support.

In addition to many other helpful topics, Linda takes on the discussion of temperament, and is able to help her readers see the connection between traits that may have fueled their eating disorder, and how these can come back into play and affect them during or after pregnancy. For example, she reminds those with common eating disorder traits such as perfectionism, a desire for control, and anxiety, that they cannot control the process during pregnancy, but that is OK. She helps readers see that although they don't get overall control, they do get to make many choices, one at a time.

By sharing her experience and her clinical wisdom, Linda helps readers; encouraging people to get information, but also to do what feels right, knowing that their experience will be personal to them.

I love that Linda does not leave out the need for a spiritual component that is unrelated to any religion or dogma but rather to the idea of connection to one's true essence. During my career as an eating disorder therapist I have promoted the idea that people with eating disorders benefit from reconnecting to what I call their soul self, their essential essence beyond the ego/mind, that is connected to the larger whole. Linda understands the importance of this connection and knows from experience that both an eating disorder and motherhood can interfere with it. In her chapter on spirituality, Linda shares helpful experiences from other moms as well as techniques for connecting with spiritual practice.

I believe that anyone with an eating disorder or an eating disorder history who is pregnant, or thinking about getting pregnant, can benefit from this book, as can the clinicians who treat them and the significant others who love them.

Carolyn Costin, MA MFT 13192
The Carolyn Costin Institute
Training Eating Disorder Clinicians and Coaches
Carolyncostin.com

Acknowledgments

— ♡ —

It takes a village to raise a child…and a book.

Like many authors, I wrote this book because it was the book I wished I had. I wrote it so it will now be there (here) for other new moms in need. However, the book was not raised alone. In fact, like my own recovery 20 years ago, the book began to thrive, grow, and develop when I reached out to others for support.

Leslie Keenan was a "recovery mama" for this book from the first trimester. She helped nurture it – and me – through this book's entire pregnancy, labor, and delivery. Julia McNeal is an editor extraordinaire. She not only corrects 3009 sentences while keeping the original feel, tone, and meaning, but she does it while cheerleading you on, in her own authentic voice. Jennifer Kreatsoulas assisted with editing – and believing in – this book from its early stages. She also graciously agreed to share her experience and hope in Chapter 8, Spirituality, Recovery, and Motherhood. Brooke Warner assisted with the book proposal editing, for which I am grateful.

Berni Xiong (that's Berni with no e) is the most compassionate, energetic, and go-getting "shin kicker" of a coach (writer, entrepreneur) I have ever met. She is truly a book midwife: she gets right in there with the bloody mess of it and helps you emerge with a beautiful baby. Michelle Olsen: you rock. Steadfast, consistent, compassionate, warrior, mommypreneur, friend. Shannon Meyers, MFT, helped me survive and thrive through my own journey of pregnancy and postpartum, for which I will be forever grateful. Thursday people – Lisa, Terra, Lisa Maria, Sheira, Teya, Elizabeth, Marilyn, Kristin, Sharon, Cynthia, Julia – you are the lifeboat to sanity. Thanks for modeling "You can't keep it unless you give it away, but you can't give it away unless you have it."

So many of my expert colleagues agreed to be interviewed for this book in order to share their wisdom: Sheira Kahn, MFT; Dr. Angelique Millette; Lindsay Stenovec, RD, CEDS; Leora Harling, MFT; Jennifer Suffin, IBCLC; Britt Fohrman, doula; Crystal Karges, RD. Many others – therapist moms, recovering moms – contributed their experience anonymously so that other recovering moms would know they are not alone and there is hope. Carolyn Costin, MA, MEd, LMFT, CEDS, FAED, rose to the invitation of writing the foreword with grace and passion. *Thank you.*

Jonathan, LOML, without whom I might still be in the not-choosing-to-be-a-mom camp, believed in this book baby like he believed – and believes – in our baby. Thank you, Hon. Of course the publisher is in London. We can't have an American book if we have a half-Brit child.

LOML Jr., Mr. AJWSK, thank you for choosing me to be your mom and for writing morning pages right alongside me for the past seven years. They started out as scribbles and now they are complete sentences. Keep growing. You are a miracle. You are the miracle I didn't think was possible. *I love you to the moon and back, plus infinity. (Times infinity. Plus 46.) Always – in all ways – and forever.*

I am so very grateful to Jessica Kingsley for publishing "books that make a difference," and believing in this one.

Abbreviations

——— ♡ ———

BED – binge eating disorder

BMI – body mass index

DBT – dialectical behavioral therapy

HAES – Health at Every Size®

IBCLC – International Board Certified Lactation Consultant

IVF – in vitro fertilization

LGA – large for gestational age

LOML – love of my life

MDD – major depressive disorder

MFT – marriage and family therapist

NICU – neonatal intensive care unit

OCD – obsessive compulsive disorder

PMAD – perinatal mood disorder

PPD – postpartum depression

REM – rapid eye movement

SAHM – stay-at-home mom

SGA – small for gestational age

SIDS – sudden infant death syndrome

Introduction and Overview

——— ♡ ———

Eating disorder recovery and new motherhood are both rites of passage that require time, compassionate and curious attention, and lots of trial and error to shift into mastery. Many new moms and women in early eating disorder recovery say, "No one told me that: no one told me how hard it would be, no one told me about all the physical and emotional discomfort! No one told me the ways these changes would impact every aspect of my life and my identity! No one told me it isn't about having or attempting to have the perfect post-baby body or bounce easily back into my old self!" Well, I'm here to tell you: your old self is gone. Regardless of whether you embrace it or not, it is gone. This can be the good news, the bad news, or just the news.

The three events that have been the most difficult, the most life-changing, and the most transformative in my own life have been:

- recovering from an eating disorder
- earning my doctoral degree and licensure as a clinical psychologist
- having a baby.

My eating disorder recovery prepared me to be present, and to know the terrain, in order to be of service for others in the recovery process.

Earning my doctoral degree in psychology and working in the recovery/ mental health field for 13 years prior to becoming a parent prepared me to open a psychotherapy practice specializing in women's recovery. But none of these prepared me (very much) for having a baby.

I remember one moment in very early motherhood, in the midst of the sleep-deprived haze, going for a walk along the beach with new babe attached to me. I was in the first six months, and my third (yes, third) bout of mastitis. I called a friend who was also a mom recovered from an eating disorder and said, "I can't believe *all* mothers go through this! How do any of us survive? How is it that there is no training to prepare us for this?"

Pregnancy and early motherhood are surprisingly similar to early eating disorder recovery. The changes in body size, body image, identity, changes in hormones, mood, sleep, changes in eating, the distress of being with new learning challenges, the dangers of isolation and perfectionism, and the need for support are all similar. Questions about "work–life balance" (note the quotes: I have not yet found a mom who has truly been able to accomplish this) also raise significantly similar challenges. I will introduce all of these topics here. I will then explore, chapter by chapter, each of them, more fully.

Chapter 1: Body Image

Just like in early recovery, changes in weight and/or not feeling in control of the size of your body can be emotionally distressing. When I was pregnant, people would frequently say to me, "You look radiant!" And I thought, *"F*ck you. I feel like a walking hippo-whale!"* But, after 15 years of recovery, I had developed enough skills to be able to graciously receive compliments without restricting/avoiding them (anorexia) or deflecting/throwing them up (bulimia). I also realized, as I often tell my clients, fat (or feeling like a hippo-whale) is not a feeling.

For someone recovering from an eating disorder, fear of "fat" masks underlying feelings such as fear, anger, grief, shame, vulnerability, and insecurity. I tell my clients FAT = Feelings Are Thick. When approaching the threshold of becoming a mom, feelings of uncertainty, vulnerability, fear, and insecurity grow large. Feelings of shame, under the judgment that "I really should be over this body image thing by now," are also common. But most women struggle, in some capacity, with the drastic changes to their body after giving birth.

The reality of a postpartum body is: your stomach will never be the same. This can be a source of pride (a baby grew in there!), ambivalence (I love my baby, but not my stomach), or distress (where did my body go?). Add this ambivalence to Western media culture's unwillingness to print and portray actual women's bodies in all of their shapes, sizes, and ages, along with the roller coaster of perinatal (the term "perinatal" refers to the time during pregnancy and postpartum) hormones...and a culture of body-hatred is born for moms. How to cope with, talk back to, and transform this body-hatred will be explored in this chapter.

Chapter 2: Postpartum Depression and Perinatal Mood Disorders

Fear of infertility and the desire to have children can be a motivating factor to recover from an eating disorder. And yet research shows women with a history of eating disorders tend to have more symptoms of anxiety and depression compared to pregnant women without eating disorders.[1] The stresses of pregnancy and postpartum can exacerbate the challenges of recovery and contribute to the development of a perinatal mood disorder. Despite some women's hopes, pregnancy – and becoming a mother – does *not* cure an eating disorder.

Postpartum depression is the number-one complication of childbirth.[2] Research shows that up to 21 percent of women are affected by a perinatal mood disorder during pregnancy or postpartum.[3] Given the risk factors for women recovering from eating disorders, the percentage of women who develop a mood disorder during the perinatal period is most likely higher for this population. Perinatal mood and anxiety disorders (sometimes referred to as "PMADs") include depression, anxiety, OCD, psychosis, and other mood disorders during pregnancy and postpartum. PMADs – especially depression and anxiety – are not rare. And yet it is still common to believe that PMADS are rare. Why? The answer to this is multifaceted and includes lack of awareness of symptoms among new mothers, variability in how PMADs present, shame, and lack of screening. Many moms do not know the difference between the baby blues (which is very common for new moms) and a full-blown mood disorder. In addition, there are no universal screening programs, and many barriers to treatment. Questions about PMADs, and how they are different from the baby blues, and symptoms of mood disorders (as well as how they interact with eating disorders) will be addressed in this chapter. In addition, we will look at issues that women recovering from both eating disorders and mood disorders face, such as overcoming shame, deciding whether or not to take medication during pregnancy or breastfeeding, and how untreated postpartum depression could affect your child.

Chapter 3: Sleep

Lack of sleep and lack of quality sleep are key ingredients involved in mood disorders such as depression, anxiety, and psychosis. One study linked sleep disruptions not only to infant awakening but also to hormonal factors, which affect neurotransmitters that regulate sleep. Postpartum women with depressive symptoms experience poor sleep quality, less sleep, longer time to fall asleep, more sleep disturbance, and less time in REM sleep.[4] *Sleep is essential to good mental health, and yet, what new mom is getting enough quality sleep?*

As a new mom I definitely struggled with sleep "training," modified sleep training, chucking sleep training out the window, and co-sleeping with a baby kicking me in the face. The main thing that I needed to know during this time (despite popular wisdom: "It gets easier in 3/6/12 months") was: *You are not alone in struggling with this.* In this chapter, I interview a sleep consultant about her work with recovering women and the wisdom she has to offer. This chapter also looks at advice on sleep across the spectrum of parenting philosophies – and how there is no one right answer to how you, and your baby, can get good quality sleep.

Chapter 4: Food

All pregnant women are aware of, and potentially struggle with, special food needs during pregnancy. Avoiding foods that are contraindicated during pregnancy, avoiding alcohol, and craving specific foods are almost universal concerns during pregnancy. Women recovering from eating disorders, however, often have extra sensitivity in these areas.

For myself, I was extra hungry, during pregnancy, postpartum, and while breastfeeding. I often felt ravenous. Even after years of truly trusting my body and listening to my hunger and satiety cues, this still felt disorienting. Could I really *still* be hungry? In order to maintain my recovery, I had to ignore commonly shared "nutritional advice" offered by mainstream media, books, and non-recovering moms. As an eating disorder therapist and a recovered woman, I am an activist in the belief that no food is "bad." If you have a medical condition such as gestational diabetes, you may need to be mindful about eating in a way that supports you and your baby's wellbeing during this time. However, in eating disorder recovery, balance – not obsessive control – is the key.

You are not a "bad" or "good" person – or mother – if you eat (or don't eat) any particular food. In this chapter, I interview a dietician mom who specializes in supporting recovering moms during the perinatal period. We look at the practices of intuitive eating[5] and Health at Every Size® (HAES).[6] Among other principles, intuitive eating and HAES reject diet mentality, celebrate body diversity, challenge assumptions around weight stigma, and encourage eating in a flexible way that honors hunger and satiety. How to find balance and say no to being obsessive or disordered with food during the perinatal period will be covered in this chapter.

Chapter 5: Labor, Delivery, and Postpartum

Labor and delivery are the immense rites of passage in which you cross over the threshold into motherhood. Anticipating this threshold, therefore, often includes fear, anxiety, and worry. It is important, especially for women with a predisposition toward perfectionism, a desire for control, and anxiety, to know that you cannot control this process *and that is OK*. Not only can you not control it, you're not supposed to. If you are recovering from an eating disorder, this lack of control might be a tiny bit distressing. (If you're like me, you might send urgent messages to your pregnant belly at exactly week 40: *Time To Come Out, Baby! Now is the time! I set an alert on your calendar for you! It's time to emerge, NOW!* My baby, as I'm sure you can imagine, came out in his own sweet time.) Trying to control labor and delivery is like trying to look like Barbie when you are 5'2" with dark brown curly hair and have a (insert whatever fruit analogy you want here)-shaped body. It's just not going to happen.

You *can* make a birth plan. You can share your birth plan with your birth team (family members, ObGyn/midwife, doula). Prepare for the birth that you want. Attend birth classes, meet with doulas, practice your breathing exercises. Make it known that you would like a home birth, an epidural (or not), pain medication (or not), to be induced (or not), or have a C-section (or not). But the truth is, you are going to have the birth experience that you have. Just like recovery (and the long journey of motherhood beyond postpartum), you don't get to be in control. You get to have choices, one moment at a time. You get to choose your response to the actuality of your experience.

In addition to anxiety and a desire for control, women recovering from eating disorders have unique medical challenges to be aware of during labor and delivery, and postpartum needs. In this chapter we look at a variety of birth experiences from recovering moms as well as medical and non-medical interventions. You will hear from a doula on how she helps women prepare for their birth and postpartum recovery experience. In addition, this chapter will offer suggestions to set up support for yourself postpartum.

Chapter 6: Good Breast, Bad Breast, Good Enough Breast

Should I breastfeed? Should I supplement? What if I can't or don't want to breastfeed? I remember what a shock it was, when first meeting with birth professionals (doulas, parent education teachers, lactation consultants), to discover how hard it can be to breastfeed. I thought, "Wow, it's a miracle any of us have survived!"

The current culture is very pro-breastfeeding. I understand the World Health Organization's recommendation: "Exclusive breast-feeding is recommended up to 6 months of age, with continued breastfeeding along with appropriate complementary foods up to two years of age or beyond."[7] Among other reasons, breast milk provides optimal levels of vitamins and nutrients for your specific baby, is easily digestible, and provides antibodies against illness and infection. In this chapter you will hear from a lactation consultant on her experience of helping postpartum moms in their experiences with breastfeeding, partial breastfeeding, or transitioning out of breastfeeding. However, breastfeeding is not for everyone.

As a clinician, I see many women who have incredible difficulty breastfeeding, who need to be on medication due to perinatal mood disorders (many such medications are safe to take while breastfeeding, some are not). For many women, breastfeeding also triggers memories of sexual abuse, which makes it excruciating. Finding a way to feed (whether it be breast or bottle) without re-traumatizing themselves is essential for these women. This chapter will look at balancing feeding your baby with caring for yourself.

Being a new mom is challenging, whether you are breastfeeding, formula feeding, or partially breastfeeding and partially formula feeding. I believe that the babies do well if their *moms* are supported. This means instead of "breast is best," shifting to "fed is best." As your baby is learning to tolerate the distress of experiencing hunger, you may also experience distress in practicing being imperfect. Being good enough, even when feeling inadequate, is a learned skill. We will look at practicing being good enough in this chapter.

Chapter 7: Distress Tolerance

Distress tolerance, a term from dialectical behavioral therapy founder Marcia Lineham, can be defined as "learning to bear pain skillfully."[8] It is a concept – and practice – that borrows from the Buddhist premise that suffering is an inextricable component of life itself. Pregnancy, labor and delivery, and new motherhood pretty much guarantee you will gain experience in tolerating distress. For women with temperaments that lean toward perfectionism, high sensitivity to rejection and failure, and a low tolerance for negative affect, the perinatal period can be particularly distressing. Women with these temperamental traits (a.k.a. many women who develop eating disorders) are also at risk for isolation because they think they should figure it all out and be Supermom *before* reaching out for support.

In this chapter we will look at how tolerating distress is not the same thing as *liking* it. We will challenge the myth of the perfect Facebook/Instagram/Pinterest mom. I will encourage you: if you are going to compare and despair, then you must be fair. We will look at how you learning skills to regulate your emotions can help you regulate your baby's big feelings (or vice versa: often the baby teaches us). I will encourage you to reach for support *before* you have mastered motherhood. In this chapter, we will look at the messiness of motherhood, and how you can lower the bar on unrealistic expectations.

Chapter 8: Spirituality, Recovery, and Motherhood

I define spiritual practice as a daily practice that reconnects you with the-part-of-you-that-knows. In eating disorder recovery, some people call this your "recovery voice." There are many names for this part of the self. In 12-Step recovery programs, it is often called your "higher power." Dialectical behavioral therapy calls it "Wise Mind." Jungian therapists call it Self (with a capital S). The important part isn't the name, but the connection with it. In an interview about their book *Yoga and Eating Disorders*, Carolyn Costin and Joe Kelly state:

> discovering one's true self can mean many things to many different people, but in the context of our book, discovering one's true self means to discover oneself beyond the thinking ego/mind to a deeper essence that does not get overly caught up in things…like…possessions, money,

clothing sizes, or a number on the scale. Our true self is the witnessing presence, or soul self, that is not concerned with such things. It is the deeper essence of who we are…that is connected to the larger whole.[9]

In my training in imaginal psychology, it was called "the Friend." This part of the self is compassionately objective. It can also take different tones at different times. For example, if the critical or eating-disordered part of your self is attacking you, this part can say, with great fierceness, "*Back off!*" It also has the capacity to be a nonverbal, spacious presence, filled with love and compassion. It can have a wry or sprightly sense of humor. This deep knowing part of you is not attached to any kind of investment in looking or being a certain way. It doesn't care about the size of your postpartum body, what you eat, or whether you are wearing your baby in a sling or putting your baby in a pack-and-play. This part of the self is concerned with providing as much love to you and your baby as possible, in any given moment. In an eating disorder, and in motherhood, this connection can get easily lost.

There are many ways to connect with this part of the self: journaling, yoga, meditation, walking, deep breathing, prayer. However, it can be hard to find a time to fit these practices in with the demands of motherhood. Techniques for connecting with spiritual practice – as well as experience from a mom who has been through losing, and re-finding, this connection with her self – will be expanded on in this chapter.

Chapter 9: Stay at Home Versus Working Outside the Home

Every mom I talk with struggles with working: inside the home, outside the home, inside and outside the home! The stay-at-home moms (SAHMs) don't miss their babies' first steps, first words, and glimpses of discoveries that will never happen again. They often (but not always) have an easier time with feeling confident in secure attachment and tending to their children's growth steps. These moments are priceless. SAHMs can also feel bored out of their minds and somewhat unfulfilled. Who wouldn't be, spending entire days with preverbal companions making stinky poop? Maternal ambivalence is an unspoken epidemic, due to the myth that motherhood is glowing and delivers all of your unfulfilled desires.[10] Staying home is not the right choice for every mom and not a viable choice for every mom. Some moms, like myself, enjoy working outside the home and love their professions as well as caring for their child/ren. Some moms need to work outside the home from an economic standpoint.

Women continue to do much of the work within the home, even while working outside the home, which can feel exhausting.[11] Many of these moms also wrestle with guilt. We'll talk about that. In this chapter, I interview several moms who share their varying experiences of work.

Chapter 10: Advanced Maternal Age

Choosing to have children in later life is becoming more and more common. In developed nations, many women want to solidify their education, work, find the right partner, or do personal growth work (a.k.a. recovery) prior to having children. The Centers for Disease Control and Prevention reports:

> Delayed childbearing in the United States is evident in the 3.6-year increase in the average age at first birth… The dramatic increase in women having their first birth at the age of 35 years and over has played the largest role in the increased average age of first-time mothers… many other developed nations have observed increases in average age at first birth…[12]

Becoming pregnant over the age of 35 carries both medical risks and potential psychological advantages, which we will explore in this chapter. Becoming a parent and entering middle age are both rites of passage in a woman's life. When not honored, seen, and embraced, these transitions can turn into eating disorders and body image distress. A study published in *The International Journal of Eating Disorders* suggests that body image distress and a desire to fit a thin ideal do not diminish with age. Many women struggle with disordered eating or a full-blown eating disorder in middle age.[13]

Ageing women face cultural taboos around taking up space, speaking "too" loudly, and not being seen. They face the task of embracing aspects of beauty and wisdom that Western media is terrified of in women: wrinkles, thick middles, saggy boobs, gray hair. Middle-aged women also face stressors such as medical issues, (peri)menopause, death of a parent or a spouse, divorce, and career challenges. Issues specific to having a child at age 35 and beyond will be explored in this chapter.

In this chapter, I also interview a recovered mom who had her first child at the age of 50. She shares her experience with eating disorder recovery, relationships, losses, depression, choosing to adopt an embryo, becoming pregnant, and finally, giving birth.

Resources

Resources for issues specific to recovering women are included at the end of the book for topics such as eating and perinatal mood disorder treatment, giving birth as a trauma survivor, and partners of moms with PPD.

In Conclusion

When you become a mother, you are no longer the same person. You have a choice about how to handle your transformation: how much suffering you need to endure, and how much curiosity and compassion you bring to this change. In the words of Pema Chodron, "The central question of a warrior's training is not how we avoid uncertainty and fear but how we relate to discomfort."[14]

When I was a new mom, what helped me was referencing the experience of early eating disorder recovery: how difficult it was, and what helped me survive. I remembered the affirmations I would say when I was bone-weary tired or overwhelmed with anxiety. I remembered the importance of support, of meeting with others traveling the same journey. I remembered what one of my mentors would tell me when I was struggling with body-image obsession: "the size of your body is not your business." It was a tough-love intervention, but it kept me focused on what I *really* wanted: more than the obsession, I wanted recovery.

As a pregnant woman and new mom, I read books. Any book I could find that would potentially be a guide or a friend, addressing where I was and what I was heading into, at each stage of the journey: pregnancy, labor and delivery, new mommy-hood, breastfeeding, sleep, infant and child development, attachment, working motherhood. There are many, many prescriptive books on these topics out there. This is not that book. This is not a prescriptive book. I'm not going to tell you whether you should breastfeed, sleep-train, attachment-parent, or work outside the home. I'm not going to tell you the "right" way to deliver your baby or give you the "right" food plan. This is a book that encourages you to find and cultivate a fiercely compassionate mothering voice *inside* yourself and for yourself as you learn to parent a newborn, outside yourself.

This is a book for moms recovering or recovered from eating disorders, disordered eating, and/or body-image distress. I never found a book out there that could help me through the rite of passage of motherhood *and* eating disorder recovery.

One day, walking in the sunshine, about one year postpartum, I thought, "Wow, this has been really hard. When I finish getting through this rite of passage, I am going to help others and, hopefully, make it less hard for them."

William Stafford writes about "the thread you follow": "There is a thread you follow. It goes among things that change. But it doesn't change. People ask what you are doing. They can't see the thread… But when you hold it, you can't get lost. Don't ever let go of the thread."[15]

This book is that thread. I hope it can be a friend that is in your purse, diaper bag, by the bed/crib/bassinet/pack-and-play. Take what you can and leave the rest. Keep what is helpful. I am deliberately leaving out as much "triggering" information as possible (weight, clothing sizes, specific foods, amounts of exercise, etc.). That being said, in the pages ahead, I *will* be sharing my own experience, and the experience of colleagues, along with useful research information. This is less about the content and specifics than about the process of sharing – that someone is further along the journey and reaching back to support you in *your* choices and experience, whether or not they are the same choices and experience. If nothing else, I hope you can hold onto this thread:

Recovery is possible. You are not alone.

1
Body Image

—— ♡ ——

Navigating Changes in
Your Body and Your Identity

Body image is killer for me right now. Which is so hard, because I do this for
a living! I sometimes wish I had a different career, because I went into this
work feeling like I believed in 100 percent recovery and had healed fully all
my body-image issues…so I believed my clients could, too. And now my
body image is so painful, it makes me cry at times, so it's hard to maintain
as much hope for others.

– Eating disorder recovery therapist in her first year postpartum

My pregnant clients tell me that their number one fear is that they will
lose their pre-pregnancy body forever. They are afraid pregnant and
post-pregnant women are not attractive, loved, or valued. Here are a
few more of the (false) beliefs they struggle with, which we will explore
(and challenge) in this chapter:

- There is a right amount of weight to gain during pregnancy and
  a right amount (with a right timeline) to lose it, postpartum.
  If you accomplish this, you are "normal," which means happy,
  successful, competent, and confident.

- You will feel happy if you get your pre-baby body back.
- Grief should be a brief process.
- If you still have a baby bump postpartum, it's because you don't work out enough, are overeating, or both. If you look like a Victoria's Secret model, you have it all.

Maybe you struggle with some of these false beliefs. How can you calm your fears and make peace with what is happening? How can you challenge these beliefs? Speaking from experience, it takes a process of adjustment, acceptance, and some rebellion against the norm to make the transition into motherhood and your new body.

Myth: You Will Feel Happy if You Lose Weight and Get Your Pre-Baby Body Back

Before becoming pregnant, I naively assumed, like most non-mothers, that the weight you gain in pregnancy is the weight of the actual baby. In other words, I thought I would gain X amount (I am deliberately not including numbers in order not to be triggering) of weight, which I would lose as soon as the baby came out! After I became pregnant, I realized that the baby not only needs a womb-home with amniotic fluid and a placenta within to eat and grow; s/he also needs mama's blood, fluids, nutrient/fat stores, and breast tissue to increase. After the baby is born, much of that weight is still there. In fact, most women still look pregnant after giving birth! When I first heard that, the negative-body-image part of me said, *"Well, then I'm not leaving the house until I don't look pregnant anymore."* Thankfully, by then, I had 15 years of combating negative-body-image talk and could challenge it.

It is likely that your body will never be the same again after having a baby. Why should it? *You had a baby!* This knowledge can feel devastating, however, especially for moms recovering from body-image issues. One study found that affective and attitudinal body-size estimates were significantly greater in people with eating disorders.[16] Peter David Slade,[17] in his work defining body image, includes not only a perceptual component, but an attitudinal component as well. Slade discovered that while one aspect of body image (perceptual) can stay constant/undistorted, the other (attitudinal) could be distorted.[18] So you can *know* what size you are, but *feel* a completely different size. It is the fun-house mirror effect. This means that women who have a predisposition to distort body-image estimates are likely to be at risk for even greater struggles with body-image distress during pregnancy and postpartum, making the transition to motherhood even rockier than it already is.

There Is No "Normal"

Magazines are filled with articles about "the right amount of weight to gain during pregnancy," "losing the baby weight," "mommy tucks," or skinny celebrities strolling down the red carpet weeks after giving birth. Like the story of *The Great Palace of Lies* (or *The Emperor's New Clothes*), these assertions do not bear out in reality and only make us crazy. In the original "great palace lie" story, when the emperor's trustworthy officials couldn't see the cloth the swindlers were weaving (*which wasn't there*), they pretended they could.[19] Why? Because they didn't want to look stupid or unqualified. Who wants to look stupid or unqualified? And yet, motherhood, especially new motherhood, is filled with the experience of feeling unqualified. *No one is prepared.* The idea that you can be prepared (a.k.a. not have any uncomfortable feelings and/or struggle with the process of surrendering and being in a vast learning curve) is a lie. Transitions, like the transition into motherhood, are difficult, uncomfortable, and messy. The idea that weight loss will make you feel more competent/happy/qualified is a lie.

I tell my clients recovering from eating disorders: "There is no 'normal.' There is peace with you and your own unique body." There is normal *for you.* The same is true for pregnancy and postpartum. Magazines and doctors' charts show how much you "should" weigh or what is "normal." The whirlwind of information about body and weight before and after delivery can be misguided and inaccurate.

The online and in-print world is full of celebrities looking thin, glowing, or glamorous postpartum. But even they can't win: Kate Middleton was shunned for still having a baby bump after her first child was born and then shunned for looking "too good" (glowing makeup applied, perfect outfit with no more baby bump visible) just after her second baby was born. The truth is, weight and shape are just that: weight and shape. There is no right and wrong. You may or may not like parts or all of your body during this time, but it will still be the way it is.

Although I understand the medical profession's need to have empirical measurements to determine some aspects of health, I still wish weight, being weighed, and publishing "normal" pregnancy weight-gain and postpartum weight-loss numbers could be banned. As an eating disorder recovery therapist, I encourage all of my clients to be blind weighed (turn around: do *not* look at the number) at their doctor appointments. I tell my clients that scales are for fish. Your body – and your worth – are not measured by a scale. Each body, in pregnancy and postpartum, as in eating disorder recovery, *knows* its own natural weight. This doesn't come from a chart, and it certainly doesn't come from airbrushed magazine images of pregnant celebrities. It comes from listening to yourbody's hunger and satiety cues, your body's need for sleep, your body's emotions, and your body's genetic heritage. That being said (remember: there is no normal: there is only normal *for you*), your body will change in pregnancy and postpartum.

A Time for Radical Acceptance

Given that you will gain weight and change shape during pregnancy and have a different body postpartum, the challenge becomes your attitude. Can you let your deflated balloon postpartum stomach become a source of pride rather than disgust? If you feel like a hippo, can that be OK? Can you continue on with your life without giving in to the temptation to isolate your (how shall I put this tactfully?) smelly and leaky self? My personal strategy postpartum was to strap baby into a wrap and carry him over my breasts or stomach – whatever felt too scary to expose on a particular day. Not the most empowered loving-my-body strategy, but it kept me showing up to moms' groups when I would have rather hidden in the house.

This is where the recovery concept of radical acceptance can come in handy. You don't have to like your body, but accepting it will cause *so much less suffering.* Marsha Linehan, the founder of dialectical behavioral therapy (DBT), coined the term "radical acceptance."[20] It refers to completely accepting the reality of the situation in which you are experiencing discomfort – body and soul. Your body, throughout your pregnancy and postpartum, will change constantly, in its own, unique way. It can be so hard to surrender to this process! And yet, letting go of control is a huge component of pregnancy and motherhood.

You will not be the same when you become a mom. Whatever your weight and shape become afterward, *you will never be the same person you were before you had a baby.* Putting all your energy into the lie that you can be (or at least look like) the same person will only make you tired and depressed, and try to be something you're not. Here is one first-time mother's experience of radical acceptance and pride in her mom-body.

I'm incredibly impressed by what my body can do... I definitely am a little disappointed I don't fit back into my jeans, and it definitely feels like a waterbed... I don't look like a model, but I just gave birth, whatever. The actual physical way I look doesn't matter so much to me because my body just did an amazing thing.[21]

A Period of Adjustment

Anne Lamott, an author who writes about recovery, says one of the greatest "palace lies" is that grief should be gotten over quickly and privately.[22] Becoming a mother entails grief, and it takes time to "redefine" the old self and "refigure" a new one. Allow grief, allow imperfection, give yourself more time than you would have expected, and allow your body to be what and where it is right now.

Just like recovery, becoming a mom requires developing a larger and different identity, of which the body is a physical expression. Motherhood also requires actually having a different body, one that was formed to feed and nourish a child from stores of fat. Making peace with this reality requires tolerance of the unknown. In the very beginning of my eating disorder recovery, I often felt like *this is too big... I can't do this... I wish recovery were just about the food and being "fat."* Sitting with the discomfort of feelings, many of them unpleasant ones, was not fun. There is a slogan in 12-Step programs called "HALT," which stands for: *Don't get too Hungry, Angry, Lonely, or Tired.* This is hard to do in early recovery, and as a new mom, it is almost impossible. Sleep deprivation, coping with a newborn, a wailing baby, breastfeeding, and dealing with hormonal changes create an atmosphere ripe with HALTs! Since I couldn't HALT around sleep, my postpartum recovery slogan became *This is hard.* Adjusting to my new reality by creating an atmosphere within my mind of radical acceptance made it easier to relax into the difficulties of my new life.

Just like in eating disorder recovery, I was challenged to lower my expectations of what is "good enough." The perfectionistic, overachieving, self-critical temperament that served me in my eating disorder did not serve me in recovery and did not serve me in new mommy-hood. I had to lower my expectations, again and again. One of my colleagues, a highly accomplished psychotherapist, classical musician, and horse dressage teacher, gave me the wise postpartum advice to do one *small* thing each day, and that is it. And she literally meant one small thing, like one load of laundry, taking a shower, or walking around the block with the stroller. Before having a baby, I thought, *"Well, that's certainly not that ambitious. I can do much more than that."* I had also heard other mothers say how difficult it was to take a shower after having a baby. Again, I thought, *"Wow, they must be pretty low functioning. Really, what could be that difficult about taking a shower?"* After having a baby, I understood the difficulty of taking a shower and the wisdom of doing one small thing a day.

Remember, you do not have to go it alone. Ask for help, join a moms' group, get into therapy, do whatever you need to do not to be isolated in the Great Palace of Lies. Be the truth teller in your moms' group, the one who is willing to say, "I'm not feeling happy and glowing! I feel like sh*t! I want to go to the coffee shop without carrying a baby and a diaper bag full of butt cream, Cheerios, pureed carrots, three changes of clothing, two pacifiers, wipes, bibs, burp cloths, sleep sheep, and SPF50 sunscreen!" Speaking the truth of your experience can give you more comfort in your own skin than losing weight could ever offer.

More Palace Lies: If You Have a Baby Bump Postpartum, It's Because You Don't Work Out Enough, Are Overeating, or Both

Just in case you think I'm being too much of a cheerleader about acceptance here, let me share a few examples of two colleagues and therapists with over a decade each in their eating disorder recovery by the time they got pregnant. They agreed to share anonymously some of their struggles with postpartum body image.

THERAPIST #1

The really hard thing is that I feel very betrayed in some ways both by my body and by the promises of recovery. Part of what was a huge revelation and relief to me for the first 11 years of my recovery was that when I agreed to stop starving myself, my weight was actually OK. When I ate according to my hunger signals and exercised in a way that felt good, I completely lost any urge to overeat or binge, which felt like a complete miracle. I didn't feel gorgeous, but I felt accepting and grateful for where I was. Enter, pregnancy. It was hard (especially at first, when I just looked like I'd gained weight, but didn't show yet), but I got through it, telling myself that I would easily lose weight afterwards if I just trusted my body. And I did trust it. But here is what happened: I have lost no weight since having this baby. I do not understand, it makes no sense, feels unfair, feels horrifying, and so out of my control. Especially because I feel like I see the message everywhere in our culture that if you don't lose weight after pregnancy it is because you are eating unhealthily and don't have time to exercise. Not true for me. I haven't overeaten at all. I also exercise almost every day. And still haven't lost a pound.

And yet, I also see how the work I do is what keeps me going, keeps reminding me on the days I feel I cannot bear to accept that this is my body, that I am so much more than my body, that what I truly believe is that focusing on meaning and truth can heal, that my body is not an indicator of my goodness, and even, in moments, that my body is a beautiful reflection of the fact that I brought my daughter into this world. And the big gift recovery has given me is that my body-image struggles have not led to me going back to my eating disorder, which is amazing. I am committed to a sane way of eating for the rest of my life.

THERAPIST #2

Soon after my baby's first birthday, my husband and I went to Hawaii. I wore a bikini. This is significant in that I didn't wear a bathing suit for the first ten years of my recovery due to shame/body-image discomfort. And, when I did consider it, shame still held me back, as I had been taught that bikinis were for sluts or women who shamelessly flaunted their bodies. However, at 12 months postpartum, I truly did not care. I didn't even try on the bikini I had (which I had recovered enough to have worn in my pre-baby days). I just thought, "Well, if I can actually get to the pool or ocean and be able to swim or lay in the sun while taking care of baby, *great*. It may or may not happen. I'll bring it just in case and trust it fits." Ironically, my postpartum body ended up being different than my pre-baby body in a way that culturally matched what is aspired to. Due to breastfeeding, I had lost the baby weight and my breastfeeding boobs actually resembled Victoria's Secret boobs. This was an interesting thought I had, in passing by the hotel elevator mirrors in my beach clothing while pushing baby along in beach stroller: "Wow, I look kind of like a Victoria's Secret model!"

Soon after that thought I noticed and confirmed that *nothing was different in terms of my feelings or experience in the world with a different body*. I still felt tired (more so). I still felt insecure and obsessive; it was just directed more around being a good mom rather than having a less-than-perfect body. What a crock of sh*t the message is that if you look like a Victoria's Secret model, you will have everything/feel confident/be accomplished/desirable. I had "everything" in this sense and felt the most exhausted and the least desirable/confident I have ever felt in my entire life!

When a Mother's Body Is Beautiful

In my work with women recovering from eating disorders and negative body image, it is interesting to notice what body parts women tend to dislike the most. It is often their stomach, breasts, thighs, and butt. These are the areas that gain weight when becoming pregnant and a mother. Anyone who has ever looked at an image of the Venus de Willendorf (a goddess statue estimated to have been made around 30,000 BCE, near Willendorf, Austria) and thought she was fat would do well to look at a pregnant woman's body. I would venture to guess, in no uncertain terms, that goddess is pregnant! And her fertility, the parts of her body that celebrate her womanhood and the mysterious power to grow a child and feed that baby from her own flesh, is being gloriously celebrated.

What has happened to a culture that denigrates this power in a woman's body to the point of glamorizing anorexic models, airbrushing the fat out of images of women's bodies, and glorifying actresses that lose the baby weight within weeks of having a child? Not only do media images inaccurately portray the reality of women's bodies in all their varying shapes, sizes, skin tones, and degrees of wrinkles, they also deny the full range of women's emotions, life-roles, and the challenges that come with the new identity of motherhood.

In Conclusion

I have heard the metaphor that getting into recovery requires getting down on your knees to crawl through a very small doorway (the humility of letting go of your old identity). However, once you are through that door, you arrive in a spacious cathedral (your new, right-sized, larger self). I have found this to be true in motherhood as well. As in recovery, happiness in motherhood doesn't have anything to do with the size of your body. It has to do with learning to tolerate uncomfortable emotions, not only in yourself, as you become a brand-new mama, but in your baby as well! Recovery and true happiness are both about embracing a full range of emotions. And, as anyone who has spent any time with a baby can tell you, so is parenting! As you become a good mother *to yourself* by accepting all of who you are, your baby will learn how to do this too.

2

Postpartum Depression and Perinatal Mood Disorders

———— ♡ ————

How to Know When to Get Support,
Even if You Don't Feel Like It

I always thought postpartum depression was rare. I didn't realize how
common it is, and that it doesn't mean you're a bad mom. I thought it was for
moms who were so depressed they couldn't get out of bed, moms who weren't
in happy marriages, or moms who didn't care about their kids. I didn't realize
crying in the shower every day or waking up throughout the night to check
that the baby was still breathing wasn't normal.

– First-time mom, PPD survivor

A Few of My Own Memories

I can remember sitting in the car outside my home after a few precious
hours away, by myself, and thinking, *"I don't want to go back in there. I*
just want to sit in this quiet car." Immediately after that thought, I felt
tremendous waves of guilt and remorse.

Another time, well into my postpartum journey, I was walking outside with my little one. I noticed I felt different. I thought to myself, "Oh. I feel **OK**. Here's my **self**. The world is starting to feel OK again. I wish I had known that was possible. I really didn't trust that was possible."

All new moms go through a massive identity transformation during the early stages of motherhood. What's different about perinatal mood disorders (such as depression and anxiety) is that moms going through these can lose sight of getting any semblance of their "self" back.

Who Suffers from Postpartum Depression?

Despite the myth/stigmatization that PPD is a major mental illness that only affects a few severely mentally disturbed women, PPD does not discriminate as to whom it affects. It includes women in happy marriages, unhappy marriages, with difficult births and not difficult births, high-income women, low-income women, women with mental health training, women with *and without* a previous history of depression. One estimate states that 400,000 women in the United States suffer from PPD each year.[23]

An article in *Parenting Magazine* stressed how susceptible new parents are to depression. "From pregnant women to fathers to mothers of multiples to stay-at-home moms, [new parents] experience depression at rates twice that of the general population."[24] Lots of women have PPD. Although statistics often say that one in seven mothers is affected by PPD, it has recently been cited as closer to 21.9 percent, which translates into one in five, or more.[25] Think of it this way: if everyone has a mother (which we all do), and one in five of those mothers had PPD – *one out of every five adults has a mother who had PPD.*

Most likely, it is more than one in five. Why? PPD is easily missed for many reasons. For one, healthcare visits focus more on the baby. Moms often think it is "normal" to feel so overwhelmed with new motherhood. PPD is easily missed due to the shame associated with seeking help or admitting to the possibility of struggling with depression. It is easily missed because sometimes depression shows up as irritability or anxious hypervigilance. Overachieving moms are especially at risk as they strive to uphold the myth that motherhood "should" feel glowing and fulfilling.

An Eating Disorder Is an Undiagnosed Mood Disorder

Because, as a colleague of mine says, "eating disorders are undiagnosed mood disorders," there is a high comorbidity rate with eating disorders and perinatal mood disorders. As one study revealed:

> Depressive symptoms during pregnancy and postpartum were high among women with a history of eating disorders. Both binge eating disorder (BED) and bulimia nervosa (BN) were positively associated with symptoms of postpartum depression (PPD), even when lifetime MDD was controlled... [In addition], women with BN, BED, or high Concern Over Mistakes may be at particular risk of developing PPD symptoms.[26]

Another study found comorbidity rates with a mood disorder to be 55.2 percent for anorexia, 88.0 percent for bulimia, and 83.5 percent for binge eating disorder.[27] Here's what I say to my clients: "You didn't develop an eating disorder because you're stupid. You developed an eating disorder because, in many ways, the disordered eating worked to regulate your mood! You are quite smart! Unfortunately, that is the good news and the bad news."

Why? Because disordered eating, in many ways, "medicates" your mood. Talk to anyone (I have not yet met anyone who is immune to this) who eats ice cream for comfort or a bag of crunchy chips after getting in a fight with their spouse, and they will understand. Neuroscience is now discovering what many of us have intuitively known: restricting food, eating certain foods, and bingeing/purging food changes your mood.

Anorexia and Fear

The brain of an anorexic signals that certain foods or amounts of food are dangers that will threaten his or her wellbeing. In someone with a brain predisposition to anorexia, food actually generates a "risk signal." In this system, eating less (or not eating) reduces anxiety and eating more increases anxiety.[28]

So, if you have been restricting your food, and you have trouble re-integrating eating enough food, that isn't because you are being "resistant" or "stupid." You may very well know you need to eat more and should eat more. But there is still a struggle, because of the very high levels of anxiety that are triggered by what is required to recover. As one recovering woman said:

*"I'm so f*cked up,"*

turns into

"Oh. That's just the way my brain is wired!"

There is a purpose behind this shift in thinking! When you go out to dinner with your partner, who is excited about dessert, and your anxiety starts to skyrocket, you can understand from a place that is a bit free(er) from shame and self-judgment. Whether or not you are anorexic, this kind of food-specific anxiety can be a clue that you may be struggling with anxiety in general. (More on what helps will come later in the chapter.)

Binge Eating and Pleasure

For people recovering from bingeing, overeating, or binge/purge cycles, it can be helpful to know that overeating foods that trigger dopamine – the pleasure neurotransmitter – helps relieve symptoms of depression and anxiety. In bulimia, overeating is thought to relieve dysphoria (depression) and/or anxiety, and there is an exaggerated "reward" drive to eat.[29] Since this dopamine release tends to come from sugar and/or carbohydrates, that also explains why most people will tend to binge on cookies, ice cream, pastries, chips, etc., rather than on cucumber or carrots.

If you are struggling as a pregnant or new mom with bingeing or bingeing and purging, this can help alleviate the shame and the feelings of chaotic lack of control. You are trying to help yourself regulate your mood! There are other ways to do this that may help decrease shame and address the underlying anxiety or depression, which we will look at later in this chapter. But first, let's take a closer look at perinatal mood disorders, and some ways you can recognize if you are struggling with one.

What Is Postpartum Depression and What Are PMADs?

One of the most surprising aspects for me was discovering that PPD could show up as irritability, anger, or anxiety. I know I personally never felt as bitchy as I did after becoming a mom. (Yes, I do know, from 19 years of eating disorder recovery, 16 years of working in mental health settings, and a doctorate in clinical psychology that "bitchy" is not a feeling.) After becoming a mom, my "bitch" feeling levels skyrocketed.

How does one know when feelings of irritability, anger, sadness, or loss of self-esteem are in the normal range of new mommy-hood and when they are of concern and require attention and mental health support? One way to determine what is in the range of normal baby blues and what is a perinatal mood or anxiety disorder (sometimes referred to as a PMAD) is to look at how long the symptoms have been there and how severe they are. Shoshana Bennett offers two simple criteria:[30]

1. **The symptoms last longer than two weeks.**

   PMADs (which include depression, anxiety, OCD, bipolar, psychosis, and other mood disorders), like non-perinatal mood disorders, include symptoms such as changes in appetite and sleep, loss of self-esteem, and lack of pleasure. Hormone changes are dramatic postpartum, and the baby blues are usually a result of feeling this dramatic change and resolve within two weeks. Fifty percent to 80 percent of women experience the baby blues. PMADs, however, are more persistent.

2. **The symptoms are severe enough to get in the way of normal functioning, even if they occur during the first two weeks.**

   PMADs are persistent and pervasive, and can interfere mildly or dramatically in functioning and care for yourself and your baby. If the symptoms are severe enough to get in the way of normal functioning, even if they occur during the first two weeks postpartum, it is considered to be a perinatal mood or anxiety disorder.

What Are the Symptoms and How Do They Show Up?

Following is a partial list of symptoms of postpartum depression:[31]

- Anger
- Sadness/hopelessness
- Poor concentration
- Loss of pleasure/lack of sex drive
- Fatigue and difficulty sleeping
- Low self-esteem.

The diagnosis of PPD is challenging, because changes in sleep patterns, changes in appetite, and excessive fatigue are routine for women after delivery. Who, as a new mother, *doesn't* suffer from difficulty falling or staying asleep, loss (or gain) in appetite with breastfeeding and/or hormonal changes, and having less energy and motivation to do things, in the first year postpartum? Anyone with a child under the age of one year will experience drastic changes in their weight, sleep, energy, and motivation levels during the first year of parenthood!

After becoming a mom, shame for feeling anger, irritability, and restless anxiety all became part of my daily experience. The hypervigilant aspect of an anxious depression can also be quite painful: obsessively watching the baby sleep to make sure he or she does not roll over and become at risk for SIDS, reading any and all parenting books and trying to follow the recommendations "perfectly," making all-organic baby food from scratch, or doing other "Supermom" actions deplete already depleted new moms. For moms with perfectionistic temperaments, anxiety may be more likely to show up. The following is a partial list of symptoms of perinatal anxiety or obsessive compulsive disorder:

- Racing thoughts
- Constant worry
- Disturbing or scary intrusive thoughts ("What if...?")
- Fear of being alone with your baby
- The need to check things constantly
- Panic attacks
- Lack of appetite
- Difficulty sleeping (even when baby sleeps)
- Knowing something is "not right"
- Being afraid that if you reach out for help you will be judged as a bad mom.[32]

If you recognize some or all of these symptoms in yourself, please use this as an invitation (and a directive) to seek professional support. If you are lost about where to start looking for support, please see the resource list at the end of this chapter. All mood disorders have a spectrum of severity, but *all mood disorders need treatment*. You deserve and need treatment to recover. If you have a perinatal mood disorder, it is not your fault. However, you *can* choose, with support, to recover.

A Word About Psychosis

Postpartum psychosis is rare compared with postpartum anxiety or depression and *requires immediate intervention and treatment*. According to Postpartum Support International, postpartum psychosis usually has a sudden onset within the first two weeks and occurs in one to two out of every 1000 deliveries. Symptoms can include:

- delusions or strange beliefs
- hallucinations (seeing or hearing things that aren't there)
- feeling very irritated
- hyperactivity
- decreased need for or inability to sleep
- paranoia or suspiciousness.[33]

The California Pacific Medical Center's Perinatal Mood Disorder program advises:

The symptoms of postpartum depression (PPD) – which may last from a few weeks to up to a year – may be quite intense. If you have postpartum depression, you may feel unable to take care of your baby or yourself. Daily tasks, such as dressing, cooking, and working around your home or on the job, may seem impossible. Like some women with PPD, you may feel too ashamed of your feelings to tell others, including your partner. You may be afraid that if you talk about your symptoms – which may include thoughts about harming your baby – your infant may be taken away from you. But this is not likely. With professional help, almost all women who experience PPD are able to overcome their feelings and take good care of themselves and their children. If you think you have postpartum depression, it's important to seek help as soon as possible.[34]

If you are concerned, it is important to call your nurse, triage, or mental health professional to be further assessed (you can also call 1-800-PPD-MOMS, a 24-hour hotline).

How Do I Know if I Need Medication? If I Take Medication Will It Hurt My Baby?

I am not a psychiatrist, which means I do not prescribe medication. I am a psychologist and a mom. Speaking from those points of view, the decision of whether or not to take medication can be a challenging one for mothers. First of all, there are cultural layers of judgment that make it difficult to decide to take medication. "Mother" is a powerful archetype that includes many myths that are challenged when women are in the thick of becoming one. Not all mothers experience fulfillment, joy, or ease in embracing all the transitions becoming a mother entails. Wrestling with shame around not being a "Good Mother" (selfless, non-depressed, glowing) can be a deterrent to speaking about struggling and reaching out for support.

I remember a coworker saying to me when I went back to work at a mental health facility at six months postpartum, "Oh, I would *never* do *that*" (referring to taking psychiatric medication during pregnancy or postpartum). If there is that kind of bias and stigma *at a mental health treatment facility*, imagine the level of shame new mothers who are already struggling with feeling as if they should be able to "snap out of" depression feel. In a deep clinical depression, it is extremely hard, if not impossible, to "snap out of it" or "just get some exercise or sunshine and fresh air." Add the pressure and logistical difficulty of being pregnant or having a new baby while you are trying to get out of the house, and you have added many more layers of challenge.

Brooke Shields, who suffered with PPD and was criticized for taking antidepressants as part of her recovery, states it well: "To suggest that I was wrong to take drugs to deal with my depression, and that instead I should have taken vitamins and exercised shows an utter lack of understanding about postpartum depression and childbirth in general."[35]

Here is more of her story:

> I never thought I would have postpartum depression. After two years of trying to conceive and several attempts at in vitro fertilization, I thought I would be overjoyed when my daughter, Rowan Francis, was born in the spring of 2003. But instead I felt completely overwhelmed. This baby was a stranger to me. I didn't know what to do with her. I didn't feel at all joyful. I attributed feelings of doom to simple fatigue and figured that they would eventually go away. But they didn't; in fact, they got worse.[36]

She writes about how she couldn't bear to hear the sound of her baby crying, and she wanted her baby, and herself, to disappear. Even after having suicidal thoughts, she was surprised to hear her doctor tell her she was suffering from PPD. Though she felt somewhat ambivalent about taking antidepressant medication, she credits medication and therapy as "what saved me and my family." Since coming out about her experience with PPD, she says, "I have been approached by many women who have told me their stories and thanked me for opening up about a topic that is often not discussed because of fear, shame or lack of support and information."[37]

Bless Brooke Shields for speaking out publicly about her experience to help remove the stigma of depression, and for receiving the help that is necessary for recovery. By doing so, she helped pave the way for both celebrities and everyday women to continue to speak out, dispel the shame, and recover. Many other celebrities such as Serena Williams, Alanis Morissette, Alyssa Milano, Lena Headey, Chrissy Teigen, Adele, Gwyneth Paltrow, and others have spoken up about their experience with PPD.[38] Other celebrity survivors, such as Angelina Spicer, have joined with nonprofit organizations to raise awareness about PPD.[39]

Many women also fear that taking medication while pregnant or breastfeeding may harm their baby. Dr. Hale, a clinical pharmacologist who wrote the reference book *Medications and Mother's Milk*, states:

> Although recent studies have suggested that the number of women who choose to breastfeed their infant is presently 72% and rising in the USA, the number of women who discontinue breastfeeding in order to take a medication is still significant…studies suggest that the use of medications is one of the major reasons women discontinue breastfeeding prematurely…
>
> However, the amount transferred into human milk is generally low. With only a few exceptions, the dose of the medication transferred to the infant via milk is generally far subclinical… *The pharmaceutical manufacturer's resistance to using medications in breastfeeding mothers is almost always based on legal reasons, not clinical reasons.*[40]

There are many, many factors to consider when deciding whether or not to take medication during or after your pregnancy. However, in my opinion, shame should *never* be the deciding factor. Reach out for support from your doctor, see a perinatal psychiatrist, and find a therapist who is a good fit for you.[41] It is not your fault if you are depressed, anxious, or have a perinatal mood disorder, and it *is* possible to recover. Taking strides toward your recovery is the best action you can take, not only for yourself, but also your baby.

How Does All This Fit in with Eating Disorders?

Research shows that women who have bulimia in pregnancy have more symptoms of anxiety and depression compared to pregnant women without eating disorders. They report lower self-esteem, less satisfaction with their relationship with their partner, and a higher prevalence of symptoms associated with anxiety and depression.[42]

Women who were overweight pre-pregnancy experienced a higher likelihood of MDD during pregnancy. All women with weight gains below recommended levels had a higher risk of MDD during their pregnancy, regardless of pre-pregnancy BMI.[43] Suffice it to say that, if you had or have an eating disorder, you are at higher risk of developing or having a comorbid mood disorder such as postpartum anxiety or PPD. You are more likely to experience symptoms of anxiety, depression, or OCD during your pregnancy or postpartum. As with an eating disorder, prevention and early intervention are best, but it is always possible to recover. At the end of this chapter, I will discuss what can help. But first let's look at a question many mothers have.

Will Postpartum Depression Affect My Child/Children?

PPD and other perinatal disorders (anxiety, OCD, bipolar, psychosis) can affect children in the following ways:

- Behavioral problems
- Delays in cognitive development
- Emotional problems and/or depression.

According to Zero To Three, a research-based resource for federal and state policymakers and advocates on the unique developmental needs of infants and toddlers, untreated depression can have detrimental effects on children's functioning and future outcomes. Babies that have mothers (or primary caregivers) who are depressed tend to withdraw from their caregiver. This can affect their language skills as well as physical and cognitive development. Later, as they grow, this can affect their self-control, level of aggression, peer relationships, and ability to function well in school.[44]

If you have had or are currently suffering with an eating disorder or depression, your child does have risk. But that *does not mean* they are doomed. It means that it is more important than ever that you get treatment and recovery yourself! When I attended Postpartum Support International's training on perinatal mood disorders, the message that they gave was this:

There is hope, and you are not alone.

It is possible to recover, and, in recovering yourself, you help build a more protected base from which your child can thrive and grow.

What Helps?

Here are some of the tools I found helpful in the first few years of parenting that may be helpful to you, regardless of whether you meet diagnostic criteria for PPD or not:

- **Get the right kind of support:** Psychotherapy and medication interventions as provided by a therapist and/or psychiatrist can be invaluable and necessary components to recovery from PPD. Professional support is often critical for your recovery.

Seeing your ObGyn, medical doctor, and/or a nutritionist can also be helpful for looking at how to best balance your hormones and food plan for healing. Moms' groups for postpartum women, moms' groups for women with PPD, childcare and housework help, friends, and family can all be helpful in alleviating some of the weight of new parenthood and/or depression.

Ask for the help that you need. If your spouse or other loved one expresses concern, listen to them and try not to push them away. Also, it's OK to set boundaries with people who are trying to help by offering unsolicited opinions, advice, or unhelpful "help." If you have a partner or mother-in-law who repeatedly tries to "fix" you instead of listening to you, it is OK to clarify that that's not what you need. Partners can benefit from counseling and support as well.

- **Sleep:** I know you're saying, "But that's the *problem!* I can't get any sleep! I have a *baby!*" Enlist the support of your partner, mother, or support person, or hire a night doula to help you replenish your sleep debt. The link between perinatal mood disorders such as anxiety or PPD and lack of sleep/poor sleep quality is huge. Try creating good sleep hygiene for yourself by having a consistent bedtime ritual, not using your computer/ phone in bed, and limiting or staying off caffeine.

- **Get out of the house:** Note that I wrote "Get out of the house" here, and not "Go for a walk and get some exercise." Obviously, going for a walk and getting some exercise and sunshine are helpful. But for a new mom, and a new mom struggling with depression, getting out of the house is a more realistic and difficult enough goal. It can be extremely difficult if you are facing depression and caring for a young child to get out of the house. It takes turning toward the opposite action (away from what you feel like and toward what feels insurmountably difficult) to get yourself dressed (showered and fed if you can), the baby changed and fed, all the baby gear packed, and the baby into the stroller/car seat/baby carrier/wrap and step out of the house!

If you walk half a block down the sidewalk, celebrate it! If you get to the playground or the coffee shop, it is a momentous accomplishment. The link between PPD and low vitamin D has been empirically validated, so getting some sunshine can only help.[45] If you meet up with another mom, great! If you get to the beach or park and do a mildly vigorous walk, *Woo-Hoo!* Fresh air and sunshine can work wonders to shift the claustrophobia of being inside a small house, both literally and in your brain. As a friend of mine in a 12-Step program says, "better out than in," by which she means it's better to talk about the distress than keep ruminating about it inside your own mind. There is much more room on the outside for a fresh perspective. This can be true of getting out of the house as well.

- **Find humor in and normalize the shadow side of parenting:** When I was a new mom, I suddenly discovered there is a whole world on the Internet of mommy blogs. Reading about other women's experiences helped break the isolation that went along with the difficulty of making plans when having an infant on an unpredictable schedule. I was often so tired that humor helped much more than advice. One of my most favorite humorous parenting blogs, called *Crappy Pictures*, shows cartoons of motherhood, including what it is like to (not) sleep, (try to) shop, (not be able to) have sex after having a child. The author writes about poop, food, body image, and life before and after kids, with short entries and "crappy pictures."[46]

Another favorite of mine is Jill Smokler's blog (and several books) on how motherhood is actually not easy, glowing, intuitive, and fulfilling. She challenges myths of the glowing, natural (non-depressed) mother, and how "motherhood comes naturally."[47] She has a confession board on her blog where moms can write what they are most afraid to admit. Apparently, she also suffered from undiagnosed PPD.[48]

- **Be discerning about what you expose yourself to:** One PPD blog recommends that new moms stay away from depressing or scary movies, books, literature, or news.[49] This is wise advice. I would add social media to this list. Be discerning about your media exposure, or you may want to take a break for a period of time. Obviously, you can't avoid being exposed to all suffering. Suffering and violence do occur and are occurring. If you have the energy, by all means, (especially if you are living in America post-2016), do social justice work you believe in – fight to keep refugee families together, march for women's rights and maternal mental health coverage, help get people to the polls to vote, lift up women of color, and volunteer to help hurricane and wildfire victims. However, if you do not have the energy right now, know that others are carrying the torch for you. We will pass the baton whenever you are ready – but don't take the baton before you get your strength back. Putting yourself in the direct line of suffering when you are in a major depressive episode and don't have the energy to spare is not beneficial to anyone.

When we had a new baby, my husband and I watched the film *Life Is Beautiful*. This isn't necessarily a depressing movie (considering the context – *it is about the Holocaust*). Before kids, I would have thought, "What an interesting but disturbing movie," and then gone on with my life. However, seeing a father trying to protect his young son from the horrors of the Holocaust, with sleep deprivation, a new baby boy, and some disturbing similarities in the current world environment, I found myself wracked with sobbing, doubled over, unable to breathe. I couldn't make it through the movie.

There will be times in your life to watch movies or read biographies on addiction, genocide, madness, eating disorders, Holocaust survival, and emergency-room dramas. And there will be times when you will need or choose to take direct action on alleviating suffering. There will be times to actively be of service, in a big way, for others in the world. If you are a sensitive soul, and struggling in the trenches with PPD, start with you.

In Conclusion

Thomas Moore, author of *Care of the Soul*, offers the wise suggestion of simply listening to depression, to what it has to say, to what teaching it has to offer, to what needs the soul has in the emptiness:

> Because of its painful emptiness, it is often tempting to look for a way out of depression... But maybe we have to broaden our vision and see that feelings of emptiness, the loss of familiar understandings and structures in life, and the vanishing of enthusiasm, even though they seem negative, are elements that can be appropriated and used to give fresh life and imagination... Care of the soul doesn't mean wallowing in the symptom, but it does mean trying to learn from depression what qualities the soul needs.[50]

If you have PPD, anxiety, or another perinatal mood disorder, or if you are in exhausted-new-mommy boot camp, consider that your vulnerability is actually your greatest gift. Consider that the emptiness is the way out. Reach out for support. I'm going to remind you again: *You are not alone, and recovery is possible.* There is always hope, even if you need to let someone else hold it for you. We who have crossed the threshold of motherhood before you, survived and thrived, are holding the hope for you, until you can hold it again. I promise you: it will return. You will hold hope again. The way out is through.

Helpful Resources

- National Postpartum Depression Hotline: +1 (800) PPD MOMS
- Suicide Prevention & Crisis Hotline: +1 (415) 499 1100. It is important for women who might be experiencing suicidal thoughts/ideas/plans to call this number.
- Postpartum Stress Center: http://postpartumstress.com/helpful-links
- Postpartum Support International: www.postpartum.net
- MotherToBaby: https://mothertobaby.org. MotherToBaby provides evidence-based information about medications and other exposures during pregnancy and while breastfeeding.

Further resources on perinatal mood disorder recovery, including resources outside the US, are provided at the end of the book.

3
Sleep

————— ♡ —————

Life Will Never Be the Same, but You Can Get
Support and Create New Structures

I started working outside the home when my baby was three months old. A few times I think I actually fell asleep standing up. Last week my colleague was whining about how she was tired from her weekend and didn't sleep well the night before. This was a non-mom. I gave her a withering stare. She sheepishly added, "Oops. Sorry, new mom."

– Mother of a six-month-old

There is a reason why sleep deprivation is used as a form of torture. In the beginning of a cycle of sleep deprivation, there are difficulties in concentration, and irritability. With further deprivation come problems with reading and speaking, and an increase in appetite. If the deprivation continues, disorientation, visual hallucinations, social withdrawal and/or challenges, memory lapses, and breaks in reality occur.[51]

For those of us recovering from disordered eating, we may not have realized we had a sleep problem until we got into recovery. Having difficulty getting to sleep or staying asleep, or waking early are issues that often arise after we have stopped the eating disorder behaviors. When you stop "medicating" your mood with (or without) food, it can suddenly become distressingly clear how anxious thoughts wake you up in the middle of the night, or at 5 o'clock every morning. Or you may notice your tendency to oversleep and have trouble getting out of bed in the morning. You may notice you have difficulty winding down at night or find yourself in bed ruminating.

The symptoms of people struggling with sleep deprivation include impaired concentration, impaired memory, decreased ability to accomplish daily tasks, and decreased enjoyment of interpersonal relationships. Importantly, most of these variables show an increasing degree of impairment with greater frequency of sleep disturbance.[52]

Interrupted Sleep Is as Bad *or Worse* than Not Sleeping

One study, led by a Johns Hopkins University School of Medicine researcher, found that awakening several times throughout the night is more detrimental to people's positive moods than getting the same shortened amount of sleep without interruption.[53] I do not imagine that any new mom needed this study to know this. So, as we recovered from disordered eating, many of us approached new motherhood with trepidation, as we faced the reality of having a newborn, and therefore the reality of not sleeping. I remember sitting in the Post-partum Support International conference and seeing the presenter flash a slide of an infant's face looking contemplative and concerned. The caption read:

How to put this... You will never "sleep in" again.

Sleep deprivation is a reality of new motherhood, regardless of whether your baby is a "good sleeper" or not. And for moms with a predisposition toward sleep difficulty prior to motherhood, it can be especially challenging. One criterion interesting to note that differentiates infant sleep challenges from the mother's sleep challenges is that if mom can't sleep *even when the baby is sleeping*, then there is the possibility of perinatal anxiety. Moms with perinatal anxiety (or OCD) often struggle with a hypervigilant, obsessive worry. These moms may lie awake fearful about the baby's sleep, ruminating about specific details regarding the baby's wellbeing, even when the baby is healthy and sleeping. They may also experience intrusive thoughts. (If you notice this to be true for yourself, please seek out support from a therapist trained in perinatal mood disorders.)

As a new mom, I definitely struggled with sleep: "sleep training" my baby, modified sleep training, no sleep training, chucking sleep training out the window, co-sleeping with a baby kicking me in the face, etc. When I tried a modified "cry it out" approach (letting the baby cry and finally get to sleep on his own; see more below) and failed, and "hit bottom" on sleep training, I actually found peace. I chose to surrender to being flexible with what worked, one day at a time, and letting go of finding (or believing there is) a "right answer" and then beating up on myself for "failing" to find it.

The Voice of Self-Compassion

As we will see in Chapter 8, it is essential to develop and hear a voice of self-compassion inside you. Here is some of what I said to myself when I found mine:

> Lots of people have "failed" at this. You are not alone in struggling with this sleep-thing. It is OK to be angry at your husband during this phase of sleep deprivation. That is normal. Love is under the anger. (You don't have to feel or remember that right now.) I know you know a lot about the damage that can occur from inconsistent psychological conditioning, but here is what I want you to know, from a fierce mother's heart: your child is not a dog, rat, or a pigeon,

and you are not Pavlov, Skinner, Watson, or any other behavioral psychological researcher!

It is OK to be inconsistent, because you are human. One of the best lessons you can model for your child is to listen to your intuition about where you are suffering, and let that guide you toward the most appropriate response. You do not have to cut yourself off from that awareness to be a good mom. Yes, of course it can be helpful to be consistent, but remember the deeper place of consistency is the ability to flow with chaos. This is not a laboratory. This is a real-life experience with messiness and failure. And growth comes from failure. AFGOs (another f**king growth opportunity) come from failure. Remember how Brené Brown called TED "the failure conference?" There is a *lot* of inspirational growth in failure. Invite failure more! Invite yourself to fail!

The foundation of transformative learning (including recovering from an eating disorder) comes from admitting, "OK, I am not doing well, I am wholeheartedly willing to stop suffering in this way, and I want to try something different." *I invite you to wholeheartedly be willing to stop beating up on yourself* for the ways you are "failing" as a mother and embrace messy learning. As Brené Brown states, one of the greatest gifts we can teach our children is that, "You are worthy of love, belonging, and joy." And we model this for our children by modeling self-compassion and embracing our own imperfections.[54]

"Cry It Out," Co-Sleeping, and Finding Resilience with Something in Between

If you are a mom recovering from disordered eating, who has a tiny bit (or, let's be honest, a vast amount) of perfectionistic, black-and-white thinking tendencies, you might be tempted to latch onto a "solution" such as "cry it out" or other (seemingly) simple solutions to getting your baby to sleep, so you can sleep.

For some evidenced-based research and real-life clinical application on sleep, I interviewed Dr. Angelique Millette. Dr. Millette has worked with families for almost 20 years as a midwife, infant and pregnancy massage therapist, birth and postpartum doula, childbirth educator, lactation educator, parent coach, and child and family therapist. Her doctoral research addressed the various sleep choices that mothers make for their infants, and to what degree these infant sleep choices may be related to postpartum depression or anxiety. I asked her, "What obstacles do you encounter in working with moms who have perfectionistic tendencies in navigating the terrain of early motherhood and sleep?" Here's what she said:

> These moms may have a tendency to want to have sleep training wrapped up quickly, and struggle with flexibility and resiliency. If they have anxiety and a desire for control, I help them walk through creating routines and structures for the day, to create some predictability. And then I work with them on flexibility. For example, there is no science that says the baby must sleep in the crib at home for their naps. So, I work with them on, for example, having 70 percent of naps at home and 30 percent flexible (in the stroller, on the way home from mom-and-me group in the car).

Since these are the moms who are likely to isolate until they get everything "perfect" (which never happens and often leads to isolation and more anxiety and/or depression), she helps them connect with some form of support. This can include a moms' group, group therapy, individual therapy, acupuncture, doula, or other support. From experience, she knows that sleep strategies work better for families getting support. When I asked Dr. Millette about postpartum anxiety/depression and sleep, here is some of what she pointed out:

- Thirty to forty percent of the moms she saw (who are seeking sleep consulting support for their baby) have anxiety or depression.
- Moms aren't sleeping if babies aren't sleeping.
- Most of the sleep books are opinion-based, not evidence-based.

That last one, even as a licensed psychologist myself, threw me for a loop. *What?* That means that all those "sleep expert" books on the parenting shelf in the bookstore are simply different people's opinions?! No wonder they all have drastically different and contradictory advice.

Attachment-Based Co-Sleeping Versus "Cry It Out"

Have you heard of "attachment parenting" and/or "cry it out?" These two parenting methods, founded by Dr. Sears[55] and Dr. Ferber,[56] respectively, are at opposite ends of the philosophical spectrum in terms of their approach to infants and sleep. Dr. Sears is the founder of attachment parenting, whose basic premise is that mothers and babies need to be close to each other. The three basic tenets of attachment parenting are breastfeeding, co-sleeping, and baby wearing (in which babies are literally attached to their mothers in a sling). Feminist critics point out the shortcoming of this approach, which is that it basically sets up a paradigm in which you will never be good enough as a mom. As a 2012 article in *Time Magazine* points out:

Attachment parenting says that the more time babies spend in their mothers' arms, the better the chances they will turn out to be well-adjusted children. It's not a big leap from there to an inference that can send moms into a guilt-induced panic: that any time away from their baby will have lifelong negative consequences.[57]

For moms with any kind of predisposition toward anxiety, perfectionism, and guilt, practicing attachment parenting to the letter of the law can be a set-up for failure.

Attachment parenting, though founded by a pediatrician, is based more on Dr. Sears's (and his wife's) experiences than research on sleep health. Dr. Sears's wife read the book *The Continuum Concept*, about how babies in the jungle were carried more, and cried less as a result.[58] This informed Sears's attachment-parenting principles. On the positive side, Dr. Sears and his wife clearly advocate for supporting babies' natural tendencies to attach to their parents and regulate themselves through this attachment. When interviewed about his concerns about babies left to "cry it out" on their own in order to get themselves to sleep, Dr. Sears stated of these babies, "They don't laugh as spontaneously. They don't coo and babble, you know, as often. They kind of turn into pretty quiet babies. And we call it the shut-down syndrome."[59]

On the other end of the spectrum, pediatrician Richard Ferber is known for some controversial advice called "cry it out" that tells parents crying might be helpful for babies to learn how to sleep on their own. He is also known for stating babies should *not* sleep with their parents.

For two decades Richard Ferber's name has been attached to the idea that any and every child can quickly learn to sleep through the night if parents just leave them to cry alone for a few nights. Many parents swear by this so-called Ferberizing. Others consider it just short of barbaric.[60]

In addition, as Dr. Ferber himself acknowledges:

graduated extinction [a form of behavioral conditioning that teaches parents not to respond to baby's cries at night] doesn't teach children how to fall asleep on their own. Children are simply denied access to their parents and left to work it out for themselves.[61]

Recently, Dr. Ferber has clarified he only uses this so-called "Ferber method" – the approach of allowing a child to cry for longer and longer periods – for those families who want to break what Ferber calls bad sleep habits. He states:

A typical example of that is a child who is rocked to sleep; the family is sneaking them into the crib and then tip-toeing out of the room. So, when they wake up at night, lo and behold everything has been changed. Now that child is not going to be very happy with that. If the family wants the youngster sleeping in the crib by themselves, then they have to be honest with their youngster. And you put the child into the crib awake.[62]

I love how recently both of these doctors have "changed their tune" – modifying their approaches to acknowledging that one method doesn't work for everyone, and each family can find their own right balance:

there is an area where both Sears and Ferber have changed their views. Twenty years ago, the Sears were strong advocates of co-sleeping, the practice of parents and children sharing a bed. Now, Sears acknowledges that this doesn't work for everybody. Ferber once said that parents who want to co-sleep should, quote, "examine their own motivations." In his new book, he now says co-sleeping works just fine for many families.[63]

Dr. Ferber said this beautifully: "Children are very flexible. They can sleep well in many different settings and do terrifically."[64]

This flexibility through resilience and non-black-and-white thinking fits with what Dr. Millette experiences and teaches in her sleep consultation work with parents. When she started her sleep consulting work decades ago, she shares, "There were only two camps: attachment or cry it out." She had an "Aha!" moment when she realized that the attachment-based parenting approach was not research-based, and there was no one-size-fits-all method. As a feminist, it became clear to her (especially for the perfectionistic moms who were trying to do it all, failing, and blaming themselves): "Wait a minute! This has to look different. There has to be another way!"

From this place of readiness to help parenting evolve, she developed her middle-ground methods: Low/No-Cry; Interval (in which parents check in on the crying baby every certain number of minutes, as they are on their way to learning to sleep); and Chair/Mattress (where parents lie or sit next to the baby while s/he is falling asleep). Within these approaches, she develops a plan with each family, applying what works for them. She shares that the most important factors are "We don't coerce, and we move at the speed of the slowest parent."

As any mom or dad who has attempted to implement a sleep "solution" without collaborating with their spouse knows, it doesn't work! How many moms (or dads) blame themselves for failing at sleep training when their partners tell them, "Don't go in there!" as baby is crying, and they just can't do it? My husband and I both failed. And, in a reversal of typical gender stereotypes, he was even worse than me, caving at going in to pick up the crying baby at three minutes. (I think my record was seven.) So, this "moving at the pace of the slowest parent" is vital, whether you are doing the "interval" method, co-sleeping, or any other approach to sleep. Dr. Millette says it is essential to limiting conflict between the couple.

Including the temperament of the baby is essential as well. Some babies, for whatever reason, are "better" at sleeping, earlier. I say "better" because there are no "good" or "bad" babies. However, babies do have different temperaments, right from the womb. Despite what I used to believe before becoming a mom about it all being "nurture" and conditioning, "nature" absolutely does play a role in your child's sleep and temperament. I will never forget a fellow mom in my moms' group who (bless her) didn't share until all of our babies were a year old that her baby slept through the night at three months. I think if she had shared this, we probably would have collectively kicked her out of the group or forced her to trade babies for three-day increments to help us recover from our own sleep debt!

Anxious Moms, Do Not Despair!

For moms who struggle with anxiety (as well as depression and other perinatal mood disorders), sleep is essential. They need sleep in a way that works for them and their families; not a prescribed, one-size-fits-all approach. They do not need a pediatrician, a fellow mom, or anyone else who says, "You *must* do it this way." These moms are likely already obsessively and intrusively worrying about damaging their babies – to the point where *they themselves* are not sleeping.

There is a solution. The concept of "sleep hygiene" is something I work on with clients every week in my therapy practice.

Sleep Hygiene – No, It's Not a Shower

The term "sleep hygiene" refers to practices that lead to a quality night's sleep as well as daytime alertness. According to the National Sleep Foundation,[65] here is a list of suggestions for sleep hygiene:

- Limit daytime naps to 30 minutes.
- Avoid stimulants such as caffeine close to bedtime.

- Exercise in moderation (for recovering and early postpartum women this could mean *no* or *very little* exercise) to promote good-quality sleep.
- Ensure adequate exposure to natural light.
- Establish a regular relaxing bedtime routine.
- Make sure that the sleep environment is pleasant.
- Associate your bed with sleep.

I will now expand on these suggestions, as they relate to new moms.

AVOID PROLONGED PERIODS OF NAPS DURING THE DAY

I know, I know, if you are a new mom you are likely to say, "That is the only time I can get some rest!" And everyone says, "Sleep when the baby sleeps." What I would say about this is: do what works for you. If you are able to nap when the baby naps and catch up on some of your sleep, by all means do it. If it makes you more anxious or depressed, or if it interferes with you getting sleep at night, don't. You know – or you will discover – what works for you. And it may be different things at different times. That is OK.

AVOID STIMULANTS SUCH AS CAFFEINE

Alcohol too close to bedtime can interfere with sleep. It disrupts sleep in the second half of the night as the body begins to metabolize the alcohol, causing you to wake up in the middle of the night.

Now, if you are like me, you cannot survive early motherhood – or life – without coffee. Again, notice what works for you. For example, if you drink coffee, you may want to drink it only in the morning, to have as little as possible negative impact on your nighttime sleep.

EXERCISE

The general recommendation is: more vigorous exercise in the morning or afternoon; relaxing exercise, like yoga, before bed. Remember, these guidelines were put out for people in general – not new moms. So, if you need exercise, and the only time you have a sitter or a co-parent is in the evening, and you can still sleep afterward, go for it! Also, if you're not exercising right now, or if you're exercising by doing five minutes of half-hearted yoga with a postpartum belly sagging on the ground, that's fine! This compassionate and gentle approach is even more important if you have a history of exercise bulimia in which you drove yourself to exercise in a rigid, inflexible, every-day-no-matter-what kind of way. In case you haven't already discovered this, recovery and early motherhood does not lend itself to that approach. Please lower the bar for yourself and consider a five- to ten-minute walk a valid form of exercise.

ENSURE ADEQUATE EXPOSURE TO NATURAL LIGHT

Light exposure helps maintain a healthy sleep–wake cycle. Even if you can only get out of the house for five minutes, do it! Just like pediatricians often recommend vitamin D drops for infants, vitamin D can help you, too! Did you know that vitamin D is one of the best antidepressants? Low vitamin D has been linked with postpartum depression.[66] Try to get some sunshine and vitamin D, in the amount that your doctor suggests. (If you are concerned about your vitamin D levels you can have them checked by your doctor.)

ESTABLISH A REGULAR, RELAXING, BEDTIME ROUTINE

Try to avoid emotionally upsetting conversations and activities before trying to go to sleep... There was other advice here from the National Sleep Foundation that I left out because, let's be honest, you are a new parent. There are going to be emotionally upsetting conversations (most likely with your spouse or partner) and activities (most likely with baby crying). These may happen right before going to sleep. Just do the best you can with taking deep breaths and finding relaxing rituals that work for you.

Creating a nightly ritual that helps you relax before bed, however, can help your mind begin to unwind and prepare for sleep. Some simple examples include: spray some lavender on your pillow, take baths, lower the lights, drink decaf tea, rock *yourself* in the rocking chair, along with the baby.

ASSOCIATE YOUR BED WITH SLEEP

It's not a good idea to use your bed to watch TV, listen to the radio, or read, if these activities keep you up. The screen issue is a difficult one. I know many new moms who count on their phone as their saving grace for some kind of connection with sanity during 3 a.m. breastfeeds. Also, many people say reading keeps you awake, and so you shouldn't do it in bed. Reading in bed, however, was one of the few pleasures that got me through early motherhood. You need to find what works for you.

In fact, as I believe I've said *find what works for you and trust that* about a hundred times already, I'm going to invite you to bring that sentence into your heart. The whole point of this book is to invite you to remember that you can trust yourself – that wise part of you that is under all the other chatter. You will find what works for you.

In Conclusion

This is where I urge you to do a half-assed-but-good-enough job of trying *some* of the suggestions above and leaving the rest. As with anxiety, depression, and recovery, I invite you to utilize support in getting sleep for you and your little one.

I wish you a good (enough) night's sleep!

4
Food

———— ♡ ————

How to Survive Nausea, Food Cravings, and Other
Pregnancy and New-Mommy Food Challenges

I remember I had to bring snacks with me everywhere. I would eat things right before we went anywhere because I was afraid they wouldn't have what I was craving at the time. One minute I would want French fries and the next minute they would be repulsive. When we traveled internationally during my pregnancy, I threw up in the (very long) customs line. I didn't do it on purpose, but suddenly the line cleared, and we were permitted to go straight to the front!

– First-time mom

My husband jokes about how, prior to pregnancy, I would often leave a bit of food on my plate or ask if he wanted some. During pregnancy and postpartum, I developed a fierce look he came to know well that said, *"Do **not** touch my plate!"* During the postpartum period, I remember being ravenously thirsty and hungry, all the time. My rational mind would say

Didn't you just eat?

Then my body would say,

*I'm **hungry**. And **thirsty**. NOW.*

I was recovered from my eating disorder for 13 years when I got pregnant, so I had already had a lot of trial and error, discovering what worked and didn't work for me. I had settled into trusting my natural hunger and satiety cues, and my weight had settled into its natural set point. I was able to eat more on some days, less on others, depending on natural changes in activity, hunger levels, and schedule. I had learned not to freak out if my husband wanted to eat dinner at 8 p.m. and I got hungry at 5 p.m. (eat a substantial snack). I had to eat more on days that I exercised. I had come to peace with eating dessert, and de-criminalizing food from being "bad." I no longer hid in shame while I ate an entire pint of ice cream for "dinner." (Also, I no longer needed to eat an entire pint of ice cream for dinner. When ice cream was no longer forbidden, it regained its proper proportion.) If I overate, I didn't restrict or over-exercise the next day. I ate a variety of foods and food groups. I knew eating fat doesn't make you fat, butter tastes good, and carbs are not a moral issue. I had learned the importance of maintaining a clear (but flexible) structure with eating. For example, I learned I need to eat breakfast, even if I'm not hungry in the morning. I had learned that I needed to eat a *substantial* breakfast (a latte is not breakfast), if I was going to make it through until lunch without my energy crashing.

Pregnancy completely threw me off. My hunger and satiety levels, which had previously been stable and regular for years (every four hours I'd start to get hungry), suddenly became erratic. I was *famished* one moment and full/repulsed the next. Foods that had previously not been interesting suddenly became an imperative: I *must* have a hamburger. *Now.* Tonight's dinner will be olives, hummus, and oranges. Ice cream? Yes! Right now! Oh, actually, never mind, that makes me nauseous. Get that away from me. The thought of a normal breakfast made me want to throw up – and I often did (not in a bulimic way; in a morning sickness way). It was counterintuitive for me to learn that, during pregnancy, eating made the nausea calm down. Breakfast became crackers...prior to arising, in bed. Not the breakfast I had become used to, but it stopped the nausea. During the postpartum period, breastfeeding made me both famished and thirsty, in a way I'd never experienced. I remember going out to lunch with another breastfeeding mom, waiting for our food, joking that we were so famished we were tempted to lean over to our neighbor's table: "Excuse me? We're breastfeeding, and we *really* need a snack. Can we have your bread?"

All pregnant women are aware of, and may struggle with, special food needs during pregnancy. Not eating foods that could transmit listeriosis, avoiding alcohol, and having food cravings are common concerns for pregnant women. However, women recovering from eating disorders often have extra sensitivity in the area of food. It can be hard for these women to maintain their non-diet recovery in a perinatal culture filled with messages such as "Don't gain too much weight during pregnancy!" and "Lose the baby weight as soon as possible!"

As an eating disorder therapist and a recovered woman, I had to put down or simply not listen to much of the common nutritional advice on how to eat during pregnancy and postpartum, because aspects of the diet mentality contradicted recovery. Drink skim milk to lose the baby weight? No. Avoid desserts? Nope. As an eating disorder therapist, I assist women to recover from the belief that fat/carbs/sugar (fill in your "fear food" here) are "bad" and should be avoided. Also, skim milk tastes like bluish water and butter is yummy.

I often ask my clients recovering from eating disorders whether they would feed their child the way they eat in their disorder. Would you give your baby skim milk? What about Diet Coke, fat-free cheese, no-carb pasta, or toast without butter? Would you stuff her with ice cream, cookies, and chips when she was feeling angry or lonely? The answer, unequivocally, is *No*. Being kind to yourself means not acting violently toward yourself. These behaviors are aggressive and cruel. Being a good parent *to yourself* means having loving limits around not self-harming with food behaviors. Plus, skim milk tastes like gray water.

For this chapter, I interviewed Lindsay Stenovec, a master's level registered dietician nutritionist, certified eating disorder specialist, mama of two, and founder of *The Nurtured Mama* podcast. I asked Lindsay about her experience with food and her body, and what led her to becoming a dietician. She shared how her own journey led her to this area of specialty. In college, as a nutrition major, she thought she was "doing the right thing, eating healthily," when she was actually restricting herself. She thought she was being a good nutrition major, following the rules that were given in her field. She shares: "I genuinely thought there was something inherently wrong with myself in my body for not being able to adhere to these recommendations that just weren't realistic or appropriate for my body. That would send me into these cycles of struggling, disordered eating."

Here is a beautiful "Aha" moment she had in college when studying to be a dietician. She was sitting in class having a discussion about portion sizes. All of a sudden, she realized a "serving size" listed on a box is just a unit of measure. *Under no circumstances is this the right amount for everyone to eat, every time they sit down to eat that food!* Immediately, she had complete validation for how she had been struggling with trying to stick with a cereal-box recommendation! She had been feeling so hungry, thinking there was something wrong with her body. Even though the cereal box said one bowl was a "serving size," one bowl didn't fill her up. She shares that she raised her hand in the middle of class to say:

> *I just realized that this is the unit of measure, not the perfect amount everyone is supposed to eat!* This is just a unit of measure that manufacturers picked and put on the boxes. And it just helps their product look good within diet culture, but it really has nothing to do with what you need in that moment.

Everyone, including the teacher, looked at her strangely and went back to the lecture. But for her, it was a revelation. A bowl of cereal is *part* of a complete breakfast. *Not your whole breakfast.* She began to tell herself:

> *If you want to choose to have a cup of cereal, fine. But give yourself unconditional permission to eat when you get hungry an hour later.*

Once she started to experiment with this, realizing she could relax around food, it was not scary. When she was introduced to intuitive eating, it fit with her own personal experience.

> Once I realized there was this whole world of intuitive eating and "Health at Every Size®", I knew I had found my calling. People in this ideology were saying not only "It's OK to eat," but "It's OK to eat enough and enjoy it! You have permission to do this!" I realized, Oh, these are my people! There was no going back.

Intuitive eating advises listening to your body's hunger and satiety cues, as well as giving yourself unconditional permission to eat without any dietary restrictions. Intuitive eating encourages you to listen to your body, from the inside, and trust that your body will let you know when it is hungry and when it is full. It also advocates for body acceptance. Intuitive eating embraces that bodies naturally come in different shapes and sizes, and there is no one size or shape that is better.

Health at Every Size® (HAES) principles are paramount to eating disorder recovery. These principles are: weight inclusivity (all sizes and shapes are worthy of respect and not pathologizing or idealizing), health policies that improve access to care, respectful care (acknowledging bias and working to end weight discrimination, stigma, and bias), eating based on wellbeing rather than dieting, and life-enhancing movement.[67] Linda Bacon, in her book *Health at Every Size*, brought critical evidence to both the medical community and diet culture challenging weight bias. In it she posits, and proves, that dieting – and a society that rejects anyone without an impossibly thin ideal – is the problem and that health and wellbeing are accessible at all sizes.[68]

In contrast to intuitive eating (HAES) is "diet culture." Diet culture says things like: a variety of body shapes and sizes are not OK; you can't trust yourself around portions; there are "good" foods and "bad" foods. It is quite interesting to watch diet culture over the years. Grapefruits used to be the "best" diet food, then carbs were "bad," then protein (who thought of putting bacon in everything? I mean I *love* bacon as much as the next person, but chocolate chip cookies should be made with flour and butter – not bacon) was all the rage. Recently, diet culture has been stating that we should all be eating like cave people with coconut oil, coconut flour, and coconut chips. More recently I have been telling my recovering clients, "Whole 30 will *not* make you whole."

For someone recovering from an eating disorder, learning to trust your body's signals around hunger and satiety is a journey of building trust. It can literally feel like learning to surf. You may feel unstable, shaky, and get easily thrown off. But eventually you start to get your "sea legs" and begin trusting that you *can* listen to your body's cues. Your body will tell you when it is hungry, when it is full, and what it needs. And if you listen and respond accordingly, your body can be your most beloved intuitive friend, rather than an enemy to force to "shut up and stop being hungry, betraying me, or being annoyingly needy."

This journey of rebuilding trust can take time, and also can be one of the most rewarding aspects of recovery. I can listen to my body! My body is predictable in giving me cues! My body is at its natural weight and that won't fluctuate very much as long as I listen to what it needs!

But pregnancy and postpartum can throw a wrench into even the most solid recoveries. It is the ultimate test in surrendering control. There are many ways you really aren't in control of your body during pregnancy and postpartum. For women with histories of food, weight, and body-image difficulties, that doesn't sit very well. We don't surrender control easily.

What else comes up? Shame. There's a lot of shame when a mom who's in recovery experiences an increase in disordered eating. She could be in recovery for two years, ten years, fifteen years – but if she starts to realize during her perinatal journey that she's struggling, it evokes a significant amount of shame. She forgets to take into account that this is actually one of the trickiest times for recovery; that a small or large number of eating disorder behaviors and thoughts can come back into the mind and are not uncommon. The self-talk of recovering moms can be incredibly harsh. Thoughts like "I really should be over this difficulty by now," "I shouldn't be struggling," "I shouldn't need support," are common.

Here's what dietician Lindsay had to say about working with recovering moms and shame:

> This is something that a lot of women in recovery experience. It's one of the riskiest times for recovery. And it doesn't say anything about your recovery or how much work you put into it. And look, here you are reaching out for support! You have recognized what's going on. That's you taking care of yourself. This is exactly what you need to be doing!

She stresses that it's important to make sure that they know they didn't do something wrong or are not good enough in their recovery. A lot of times, disordered eating happens as a result of the hormonal changes that women experience during pregnancy/postpartum. These are big life changes. It isn't surprising that those disordered eating thoughts or coping skills come up.

When I asked Lindsay about what else comes up in working with recovering women during the perinatal time, she shared that working through body-image shame is a key piece. Understandably, there is a lot of worry around body changes during pregnancy and postpartum. Women in recovery may take a little while to open up about that. They may not want to fully express their worry, because they don't want it to be there. They don't want to be feeling this way about their bodies. They feel shame *about* feeling bad about the change in their bodies.

The most important thing to know for moms in recovery is that pregnancy/postpartum could be a risky time, and it's OK to seek support.

Talking Back to Diet Culture

Pregnant and postpartum women are constantly bombarded with diet culture and fat phobia. Pick up any magazine and you will most likely see a celebrity mom who has "lost the baby weight" in an "amazing 3 weeks!" Most moms have legitimate concerns about how their bodies will be changed by pregnancy and motherhood. However, in diet culture, the goal becomes *getting rid of* the change, rather than embracing or accepting it. In my practice, I frequently work with assisting moms on speaking up to partners, friends, and coworkers. I help them claim (in their own words) that monitoring their weight and shape during pregnancy and postpartum is:

- not the way I choose to measure my worth as a person or a mom
- not relevant (with the exception of medical complications) to my health or the health of my baby
- not your business.

But it is hard, during the perinatal period, *not* to look to the myriad articles and books, and to fellow moms for how to "eat well for baby" and/or "lose the baby weight." I asked Lindsay how she works with moms on trusting intuitive eating during the hormonal roller coaster of pregnancy and postpartum. She acknowledged women do have some changing nutritional needs during the pregnancy period. However, they are oftentimes presented in a way that reinforces diet culture. How do we incorporate these changing needs into *our own bodies'* wisdom? For example, in the first trimester, the body is often in survival mode for many women who have pregnancy nausea. The cues from your body are so strong, they are very chaotic, and they are not to be messed with.

Lindsay shares:

> If I were to say, "Hey, you know you should really eat more broccoli during your first trimester, because vitamin C is very important, and broccoli has lots of vitamin C," and then you go home and you can't even look at broccoli because you're going to be sick, that nutrition information is not that helpful for you!

She offers, instead, something like "Oh, you got this piece of nutrition information. Let's look at whether it's supportive or not supportive to you, and how we could use it in a way that honors what your body is telling you right now." Since vitamin C might be important, there are more flexible options, such as taking a vitamin supplement during that time. And, in the meantime, you might be eating saltines and apples. The cues from your body are strong during pregnancy. You have to go with the flow of what your body is asking for.

This level of intuitive eating – of listening to your body's cues – can be very scary, or it can be very empowering. Lindsay recommends "gentle nutrition." She looks at the different stages a woman is at, and honors that healthy eating doesn't mean rigidity. Healthy eating doesn't mean restriction, or not allowing yourself to enjoy food. She urges women to know:

> *There is no such thing as a right way to intuitively eat.* There's only listening to your body and going by what it needs. Your body does have wisdom, and it is going to be giving you different information every day. And the only way you're going to know what it needs is to pay attention to it and do the best that you can.

How Can I Prevent My Own Child from Developing an Eating Disorder?

This is the million-dollar question I hear every week from moms with whom I work. The short answer? Eating disorders have a complex etiology, including genetics and temperament (which are out of your control), as well as family-system dynamics, cultural dynamics, and trauma. And so, the short answer is "It's complicated." The longer answer: genetics and temperament both *play a strong role* in the possibility of depression or an eating disorder developing, *but they do not determine it*. The hopeful answer: even if your child develops an eating disorder or depression, it is absolutely possible to recover.

The question I suggest asking is this: How can I build *protective* factors for my child? I say this because so many women blame themselves for their own eating disorder, or their child's eating disorder, and nothing helpful comes from the blame game. (Important note: If you are a survivor of abuse, it is *vital* that you do not blame yourself, and that you do trauma-specific recovery work with a professional.) You can build protective factors in your child by modeling your own non-eating-disordered relationship with your body and feelings.

My own mom spent years dieting – and then blaming herself for the eating disorder I developed later. However, she also did her own work around developing intuitive eating, thereby arresting her own dieting, as well as looking at intergenerational factors (her relationship with *her* mom) that contributed to emotional patterns that affected me. When I returned to visit my mom, as an adult in early recovery, stating, "I'm angry! And I'm not restricting my diet anymore!" we were able to talk about it. This spoke to both my willingness to do the difficult but rewarding work of recovery, and her willingness to allow me to individuate without "making it about her." And, our conversation allowed us both to continue on our own journeys.

If you're blaming yourself – or your mom – stop it. Stop blaming and shaming, as much as you can, and start practicing accountability for yourself now. *It is always possible to recover, and it is always possible to break the generational chains of suffering in your family system.* Eating disorders develop as a combination of genetic vulnerability combined with temperamental traits and a facilitating environment. Some (but not all) of the risk factors from childhood that can contribute to developing an eating disorder as an adult include: dieting as a child, having a mother who diets (or has an eating disorder), being teased or bullied, engaging in sports that are focused on appearance or weight, early menstruation, and a history of abuse.

Along with genetic links being discovered with both anorexia and binge eating, certain temperament traits tend to foster the birth of an eating disorder. The following temperament traits are often discussed among women at risk of developing an eating disorder: low tolerance of uncertainty, low sensitivity to stress/distress, perfectionism, anxiety, error detection, and harm avoidance, among others.[69]

In other words, if you have a sensitive child who struggles with tolerating "distressing" feelings such as sadness, anger, or shame, and you (or a family member) struggle with depression, anxiety, or OCD, the ground is fertile for the seed of an eating disorder to sprout. However, *doing your own recovery, and building strong attachment with your child, can help with prevention.*

I recently had the privilege of sitting on Dr. Rosanna Franklin's dissertation committee. Dr. Franklin researched maternal intuitive eating and how this can prevent children from developing disordered eating.[70] Three of the most fascinating clinical implications of the research were:

- Mothers can learn about how they can indirectly influence their child's self-regulation via body acceptance messages.
- Body appreciation is a predictor of intuitive eating.
- Body acceptance messages from mothers predict awareness of the internal feelings and functions of the body.

In other words, the more *you*, as a mother, listen to *your own* body and hunger cues, the more you *appreciate* and *do not criticize* your own body, the more this translates to your child(ren).

In contrast, a review of the literature on parent–child feeding strategies found direct correlation between parents restricting foods for their child (e.g. limiting access to snack food) with increased eating/weight status as well as decreased connection with internal hunger and satiety cues. In addition, prompts (e.g. "eat your vegetables") were negatively correlated with the amount eaten.[71]

Yep, that means not pressuring your child to finish what's on their plate, and not micromanaging how much sugar your child eats at various birthday parties. I know, it's hard! I'm on the journey with you, Mama – trusting that at *some* point in his lifetime my child will eat a vegetable. And I can model eating vegetables (and pizza, and cake) along the way.

Infants and toddlers have the capacity to self-regulate their eating given the right conditions.[72] The right conditions being: provide a wide variety of nutrient-dense food while allowing the child autonomy to choose which of these foods to eat, and when they are hungry.

Ellyn Satter's work[73] summarizes how parents can think about and put into practice modeling/trusting intuitive eating with children (while surrendering battles for control over two-year-olds refusing to eat broccoli). She defines the "division of responsibility" for parents with infants to be: the parents determine *what* the infant eats, and the infant determines *how much* she eats. She then goes on to clarify the division of responsibility for toddlerhood through adolescence to be: the parent is responsible for *what, whether, and where* and the child is responsible for *how much* and *whether* to eat.[74]

What Can I Do?

Here are five things you can do (and some you can be conscious of *not* doing) to assist with building protective factors for your child to not develop an eating disorder:

1. **Don't diet.**
   Diets don't work. This has been proven again and again. Here are a few scary statistics:
   - Ninety-five percent of all dieters will regain their lost weight in one to five years.[75]
   - Girls who diet frequently are 12 times as likely to binge as girls who don't diet.[76]
   - Thirty-five percent of "normal dieters" progress to pathological dieting.[77]

2. **Do eat intuitively.**
   Do the best you can with this, remembering there is no wrong way to practice intuitive eating (unless you are practicing an eating disorder, which is *not* intuitive eating!). Intuitive eating can be summarized as: relying on internal cues for hunger and satiety, eating for physiological rather than emotional reasons,

having no dietary restrictions/unconditional permission to eat, and body size acceptance.[78] Listen to your own hunger and don't restrict. Give yourself permission to enjoy eating!

3. **Take care of your own body image.**

   Be mindful that you are your child's mirror. You may be tempted to wear body-hiding clothing; I saw in a humorous newspaper a photo captioned "Mom's bathing suit just one giant, body-eclipsing ruffle."[79] In the photo, a mom is wearing a gigantic, ruffled curtain-like suit in which you can pretty much only see her head. Don't wear this. (Unless you like ruffles. Then, by all means, go with the ruffle.) Some of my recovering clients feel most comfortable wearing loosely fitting dresses; some feel more comfortable wearing tight jeans. (It is not only OK, but to be expected that you will still be wearing maternity clothes postpartum.) The point is that the clothes should be fitting you – not you fitting into the clothes. If there is a problem, it is with the clothes, not with you. Just like listening to your internal cues for hunger and satiety, listen to what clothing feels most like you. When you are being you, you are be-you-tiful. You may gaze disgustedly in the mirror at your postpartum muffin top. Postpartum body image and ageing can be brutal. However, don't allow yourself to buy into the culture's message around self-worth being tied to "getting your post-baby body back in shape."

   - Your postpartum body will never be the same shape. You grew a baby in there.

   - Your worth is bigger now.

   You have been changed by life. Try to embrace and radically accept that. Be proud of your tummy like your child is proud of theirs. You are beautiful because of the life you have lived, and your body reflects that: including all the scars, stretches, and wrinkles. A wizened tree does not Botox itself to look like a skinny leaf-sprout. Be the tree that you are.

4. **Follow the "Division of Responsibility" when feeding your child.** Briefly, in review, the division of responsibility is: The parent is responsible for *what, when, and where* you eat. The child is responsible for *how much and whether* they eat.[80]

I know it can be hard to trust that your child *will* choose to eat vegetables (or fruit, or protein, or a sandwich, or whatever else they're currently refusing). But it can and does happen. I have watched an amazing transformation in my own little one, who used to only eat anything soft and white. Now he eats broccoli! (By the way, *do* respect sensory sensitivities. If your child prefers soft texture, make soft-texture food, and *gradually, without a fight, making it fun*, introduce other textures.) Remember: *there are no bad foods*. Kids need carbs and fat, and so do you. They help you have enough energy, and they feed your brain.

5. **Allow all feelings in your family** (especially uncomfortable ones like anger, fear, and shame).

Low tolerance for negative affect has been shown to be one of the factors contributing to eating disorders. What does this mean? It means, in order to create an environment where your child will not feel they have to hide or stuff parts of themselves in order to be loved, you have to allow discomfort.

Anger is a tough one. Most people focus their anger in one direction (rage at others) or the other (blame self and stuff anger into depression). Work on expressing anger at the level of irritation, before it gets overwhelmingly big. Have weekly family meetings. If you get into a fight with your partner, make up, and show your child you have made up, so they can see people reunite after being mad at each other. When your child is mad, don't withdraw your affection. Notice: "I see you are mad. I'm going to help you. I love you even when you are mad. You can hit the pillow, but not me. I'm going to stay with you until we work this out."

Allow fear, and shame. Allow insecurity, embrace imperfection. When someone makes a mistake in our house, we say, "Yay! I made a mistake!" This is not my natural inclination. The natural inclination when we feel shame is to hide it. Sweep it under the rug, quickly! Pretend-like-you-know-what-you-are-doing-before-you-get-in-trouble-or-someone-sees-that-you-are-a-fraud! Don't do this. Turn *toward* your own and your child's imperfections and growth edges. Growing requires failing (and failing and failing) before succeeding. Support your child in practicing new skills. When your little one is learning to walk and falls down, you can say, "Hooray! Try again!" Continue to do this with yourself and your little one. Again and again.

It is possible to prevent eating disorders. And it is also possible to build strong protective factors so that if your child develops one, they can recover with more ease. Do what you can; it will make a difference. Eating disorders are complex and develop from a unique and individual interplay of many factors. They are no one's *fault*, but everyone's responsibility. Prevention and recovery are possible.

In Conclusion

If you are pregnant or postpartum now, I want to encourage you to reach out for support with any shame or struggles you are having. Find a dietician and/or therapist near you who specializes in eating disorder recovery and intuitive eating. Remember what Brené Brown says about shame: "The less you talk about it, the more you got it. Shame needs three things to grow exponentially in our lives: secrecy, silence, and judgment."[81] The antidote? Empathy. By talking about your shame with someone who expresses empathy, the painful feeling cannot survive.

"Shame depends on me buying into the belief that I'm alone," says Dr. Brown.[82] Shame can't survive being out in the open. When shame realizes it is no longer alone in its secret corner, it loses its powerful force. Instead of being a source of hidden fear, it becomes the ground of transformation and rebirth. If you are shining the light on your shame, you aren't just going to be birthing your new baby – you're going to be rebirthing your own self. And by listening to your body, learning to trust its signals, feed it what it needs, when it needs it, in the right amount, you are taking good care of your new self! By treating your body with kindness – sometimes it may need to be fierce kindness, telling diet culture to f*ck off – you are practicing the *simple but not easy* task of motherhood! Keep going, Mama. You are not alone.

5
Labor, Delivery, and Postpartum

— ♡ —

Having a Plan, Updating Your Plan,
Throwing the Plan out the Window

I wish someone would have told me to loosely make "birth plans" and not hold on too tightly to your perceived idea about how everything is going to go… I would have loved to hear that even if things didn't go the way I planned, this didn't mean that there was something wrong with me or that I somehow failed or that my body was broken. I think women need to know how amazing, resilient, and strong they are for growing and birthing a miracle into the world, regardless of the method or journey in doing so.

– Crystal Karges, lactation consultant, dietician, and mother of five

When I was 39 weeks and five days (but who was counting) pregnant, I went to the mall. I don't normally go to the mall. But it was raining, and I was ready to give birth. So, I went to the mall, to walk. I walked. I ate spicy food. I did *all the things*. I tried all the suggestions people tell you to do when you are nine months pregnant and ready to go into labor. Nothing. I literally could feel baby crawl up further inside, cling to my ribcage, and say, "I'm not ready. I'm staying here, where it's comfortable. You don't get to decide."

Pregnancy, labor, and delivery, and, I hate to say it, motherhood all include a level of surrender. Just like recovery from an eating disorder, you have to surrender the battle for control. You might say, but what about my plan? What about the questions I have in preparing to give birth and become a mother? We'll get to the birth plan. Birth plans are important. But the questions you have are even more important. Pam England, in her book *Birthing from Within*, writes about the questions. She writes:

> For each woman, the most important thing she needs to know will be different. I would encourage a mother to ask herself, "What is it I need to know to give birth?" Her answer must be found within, not given her by an expert. Each mother needs to find her personal, heartfelt question... Knowing your personal question is central to birth preparation.[83]

I love how this question – and the answer to it – can only be found inside your own deep-knowing self. Just like recovery looks different for every woman, so does the labor and delivery process. For some women, recovery includes a very structured eating plan, with clear, loving limits. For some women recovery includes less structure, more flexibility, and permission-giving. And, for many women, recovery includes some of each of these at different times in their recovery. Some women may imagine having a medication-free birth in a tub of water, and some women cannot even imagine giving birth without an epidural. Pam England writes about how women giving birth in a hospital need to have two different kinds of knowing: "The first and most basic is *primordial* knowing, that innate capability which modern women have but must rediscover (and trust). The second kind is *modern* knowing: being savvy about the medical and hospital culture and how to give birth within it."[84]

As a doula, Britt Fohrman is someone who guides mothers through the process of preparing for – and traveling through – labor, delivery, and postpartum.[85] Britt is a birth doula, yoga teacher, and childbirth educator who works with women in the profound rite of passage of pregnancy and new motherhood. I asked her, "What questions do you ask new moms as they are preparing for giving birth?" Here was her response:

> When I first meet with pregnant moms, I ask a lot of questions – taking an in-depth inventory of who they are, what they've been through, what their fears are, what their intentions are, if there are any specific preferences around their birth experience. I ask how they feel about their care provider, how they see their partner's role, and if they're planning on having other people at their birth.
>
> If they are planning on having people (their mom, a friend) at their birth, I ask, "Why are these people invited?"
>
> Sometimes it's actually not fitting with what they want. If they want a peaceful birth, but they invited their mother with whom they don't feel comfortable, they're not aligned with their vision. What I'm looking for is where they are – and are not – aligned with their intention.
>
> I also ask how they formed the beliefs they have about birth. Did they hear about their mother's experience? Did they hear from a doctor or a midwife? If they haven't seen a birth, are they terrified because they don't know what to expect? Is what is possible different than what they already know?
>
> In all these questions, I'm hoping to help them facilitate what is most important to align with their vision of their birth experience.

I asked Britt what pregnant moms most often ask her:

> The main questions pregnant moms have for me are "What can I do to get ready for the birth?" and "How am I going to get this baby out of my vagina?"

We talk about stopping work at 36 weeks. We talk about yoga practice, childbirth education, relaxation, breathing, visualization, and helping her partner be aligned with their vision of the birth.

We also talk about her vagina – what stories are held in her vagina and her pelvis. We talk about if there has been trauma to her vagina or pelvis. We talk about if she's been able to connect to her sexual energy during pregnancy. These are areas to bring awareness.

There Are No Bad Births

Just as in eating disorder recovery food is not a moral issue, neither are birth stories. There are no "good" or "bad" foods, and you are not "good" or "bad" if you eat or don't eat them. Similarly, you are not a "bad" mom if you have an epidural or a C-section, or have a water birth. I asked one of my colleagues, Crystal Karges, registered dietician, board certified lactation consultant, and mama of five (!) about her birth stories.[86] She shared about how her recovery and motherhood journey progressed:

While I had been in recovery from my eating disorder for a few years before I had my first baby, I think I still doubted my body's capacity to birth my baby. Even though I had wanted to try to deliver naturally, I wasn't able to fully cope with the pain I was experiencing and opted for epidurals.

With all five of my babies, I delivered in a hospital setting. I had intended to have unmedicated births with all of my deliveries but ended up having an epidural with my first three babies. I was able to deliver my last two babies without any pain medication, and these were some of the most healing experiences for me, in terms of reconciling with and trusting my body to bring my baby safely into the world.

> Having an unmedicated birth allowed me the experience of being able to fully trust my body and surrender control completely, something that had been utterly foreign to me through the years spent with my eating disorder. For so long, I hated and mistrusted my body, only to witness, firsthand, the power in trusting and letting go.

I loved listening to how her birth stories, as well as her relationship with her own body, were different each time. In my own labor and delivery experience, I planned to give birth in the hospital, in case emergency medical care became necessary. As I was advanced maternal age with a medically complicated pregnancy that required bedrest, this was important to me. However, the earth-mother primordial knowing part of me also brought a doula with me to the hospital. Although I wasn't opposed to pain medication, I did want to try to have as natural a birth as possible. I did end up giving birth without pain medication.

Notice how both Crystal and I used the words "end up" in how our birth story went. After giving birth, and hearing so many mothers' actual birth stories (as opposed to birth plans), we both now know that labor and delivery can go in many directions and can change moment to moment.

Here is the birth story of another colleague of mine, Leora Fulvio, MFT, a therapist and recovered mother of two.[87]

> Though I had planned for an unmedicated birth, I was also open to the fact that if it wasn't going to happen, that was OK. My main goal was the baby. I didn't have that much agenda or plan around the birth or the birth process. Because I had a high-risk pregnancy due to blood clotting disorders and some complications with my pregnancy, I was induced at 40 weeks. The induction didn't take, and I spent many days in serious, serious painful labor without any progression.

When I hit two-and-a-half-minute-long contractions with less than ten seconds between, I was given an epidural. However, the epidural was incorrectly placed so the only thing that happened was that my legs were numb. I was unable to move at all and was still feeling every bit of my labor. At this point, I was given a spinal injection and a C-section. My induction began on a Monday night, and this was a Thursday afternoon. My second son was born quickly and easily via planned C-section, as I didn't want to go through that again. It was pretty rough.

I asked her what she says to her clients as they prepare for labor and delivery process, and here is what she said:

I tell them that they are going to be amazing but to call me when they need me, that I'll be here for them no matter what. Motherhood is different for everyone, and I never expect anyone to have a typical experience. It's atypical in nature. But getting support is imperative for everyone. Don't be ashamed or afraid to ask for help or to accept it.

In my practice I see women who chose to do home births, women who chose planned C-sections, women who had to have emergency C-sections, women who planned ahead to have an epidural and pain medication, women who didn't have a plan on whether they would have an epidural or pain medication until they decided in the midst of labor and delivery, women who worked with doulas, women who didn't work with doulas, etc.!

Every birth experience is different, as is every mom, as is every child. How you end up giving birth is not a moral issue. So many women "should" on themselves around making their idealized birth plan. Then, if it doesn't go according to plan, they blame themselves. No matter what your plan, here are some awareness factors around medical interventions and risks.

Medical Interventions

There are medical interventions that snowball on each other, once started. So, if you want to have a natural childbirth, know that each intervention makes it increasingly difficult not to continue further interventions. Routine interventions include: restrictions on eating and drinking, intravenous fluids, electronic fetal monitoring, epidurals, augmentation (amniotomy, Pitocin®, or both)[88] and episiotomy. According to some research, women who received care from midwives (compared with women who received care from an ObGyn/medical team in a hospital setting during labor and delivery process) were less likely to experience interventions and were more satisfied with their care.[89]

There are risks with medical interventions. Two risks associated with the use of Pitocin® could and epidurals are higher risk for a perinatal mood disorder (depression or anxiety) and less likelihood of breastfeeding. For women exposed to peripartum oxytocin (Pitocin®) with a history of pre-pregnancy depression or anxiety disorder, the risk of depression or anxiety increased by 36 percent and for women with no history of a mood disorder the risk increased by 32 percent.[90] Mothers are more likely to breastfeed if they had an unmedicated vaginal birth; mothers who perceived their labors to be difficult, experienced high levels of pain, or had planned or emergency C-sections were more likely to experience depressive symptoms.[91] Later in this chapter (and in Chapter 2), we explore perinatal depression and anxiety, as well as their prevention and treatment. However, first let's look at some non-medication options for labor and delivery.

Non-Medical Interventions

You probably already know and use these strategies every day with children, your friends, your spouse/partner, and, ideally, yourself in your recovery process. Touch and skin-to-skin contact have been shown to increase oxytocin (the happy, bonding hormone) and downregulate the stress response.[92] Other strategies utilized by labor and delivery nurses as well as doulas include reassurance, encouragement, praise, and explanation. Strategies used by doulas can include mirroring, acceptance, reinforcing, reframing, and debriefing.[93] There are so many ways, and so many interventions, to help you go through labor and delivery. You could have an epidural and a doula or other support praising and encouraging you. I want to emphasize again, here, for moms predispositioned to blaming and shaming themselves that (in my opinion) *there are no bad births*. If you choose to have an epidural, or if you planned a home birth and ended up having a C-section, I will not be judging you. I will be cheering you on in your entrance to new motherhood. Welcome, Mama! As much as you can, be educated and aware of the many choices and risks for the labor and delivery process. And then, get behind yourself, your choices, your plan, and your actual birth experience! (Have I mentioned that it doesn't always go according to plan?)

One important factor to keep in mind if you are recovering from an eating disorder is that you won't be "in control" during the labor and delivery process. This is not comfortable for those of us who have a desire to be in control. Your mind (the thinking, planning, worrying part) is not in charge of labor and delivery.

Here is what Crystal had to say about what she would have wanted to hear before becoming a mom:

Labor, delivery, and birth are not something that can be fully planned for or controlled. Because there is so much unknown about how our births will unfold, it feels like we have more control over the situation when we can make plans about how we want things to go. However, even the most intricate plans will not always go according to plan. I learned to maintain a sense of what I desired while also approaching my births with an open mind, knowing that there is an element outside of my control. This, too, took surrendering to my body and having faith in something greater than myself through moments of fear and uncertainty.

So, by all means, make a plan, but hold that plan loosely.
But what is a birth plan?

Birth Plans

According to the American Pregnancy Association, "The birth of your baby should be one of the most memorable, life-changing, and joyful experiences of your life. You will want to spend time thinking through the details of your hopes and desires for this special event."[94]

Most moms I know, who have already given birth, would chuckle at the wording choice of planning "the details" for this "joyful experience." I certainly wouldn't use the word "joyful" to describe labor. However, if you want to, you should write the birth plan. (This is actually a "could" not a "should." Sorry for "shoulding" on you.) Writing the plan can help with the part of you that likes to feel in control. It can also help guide you when you're too overwhelmed with pain to verbalize instructions to your partner. You can just yell something to the effect of "Did you not read the f*ing plan?!"

Don't worry. They'll forgive you later for swearing at them.

Write your plan and share it with the hospital, your midwife, your partner, your spouse, your doulas, your mom, whoever needs to be aware of your preferences. Write about who you want to be present, whether you want to have a doula or not, what you will do for pain management, if you would like immediate, skin-to-skin contact, breastfeeding, or not. For home births, write what your plans for hospital transport are, in case of emergency. There are many birth-plan templates. You can choose one that works for you.

Though it is important to think about, and plan for, the many questions about your birth preferences, it is also important to keep in mind these are preferences, not what is guaranteed to actually occur. I planned to have music during labor and had an altar with affirmations and a candle. The hospital didn't allow the candle. And during actual labor, I didn't give a flying fig about the altar or the music. I looked at the second hand on the clock. That's what I did. For *16 hours* (with occasional walkabouts) I stared at the second hand of a wall clock. For some reason, it was helpful for me. Needless to say, that was not in the birth plan.

One woman I worked with during pregnancy was obsessed with trying not to poop during labor and delivery. She was mortified thinking about the nurse seeing and having to clean up her poop. After having her baby, she not only didn't even know if she had pooped during labor and delivery, she no longer cared. Another woman I worked with planned to have a home birth and ended up having a C-section. Another woman thought she would choose to have an epidural and pain medication and ended up not having either.

A friend of mine, who is 20 years recovered, is fond of quoting two somewhat contradictory slogans:

How to make God laugh: make a plan!

and

To fail to plan is to plan to fail.

Making a birth plan, like your recovery, should strike the right balance between these two.

Another aspect to keep in mind if you are recovering from an eating disorder is possible medical risks specific to recovering women.

Risks for Women Who Have (a History of) an Eating Disorder

Eating disorders are associated with many possible birth-outcome risks, including babies with a low birth weight or that are small for gestational age (SGA) or large for gestational age (LGA). Women with disordered eating have been found to have a higher risk of induction, be in need of assistance with breech presentation, and be at a higher risk for Cesarean section.[95]

Another large cohort study of women found that women with bulimia nervosa had a higher likelihood of miscarriage. Women with current symptoms, or histories of, eating disorders have also been shown to be at risk for low birth weight babies, intrauterine growth restriction, and premature labor.[96]

The main risk, in my opinion, and as alluded to earlier, is relapse: relapse into the eating disorder and relapse into, or development of, perinatal anxiety or depression. Research suggests that rapid hormonal changes, sleep deprivation, and the pressure of coping with a newborn cause many women to relapse into disordered eating. Here's an interesting sentence from the research: "Reversion to unhealthy eating practices is thought to be a direct response to feeling out of control."[97]

Note that the eating disorder is a *response to* feeling out of control. So, it's not the out-of-control that's the problem – or the risk. It's the response to feeling out of control. An anxiety disorder or depression can also be a response to feeling out of control. Women who have or have had eating disorders are also more likely to have had a mood disorder such as anxiety or depression prior to pregnancy. This increases the risk factor for postpartum mood disorder and difficulty with mother and baby bonding.[98]

A Word about Maternal Anxiety

Let's unpack this further, from less of a research perspective and more of a recovery perspective. As a therapist, when I consider these eating disorder relapse risks, I think about *what purpose the eating disorder is serving* and how to address that differently. You may say, *"My eating disorder isn't serving any purpose except harming me, filling me with shame, and hurting my baby and I want it to be gone."* Or you may, in your recovery process, have developed a bit more compassionate curiosity about how engaging in disordered eating behaviors "helps" an underlying need (until it doesn't any more). When the suffering of the eating disorder becomes greater than the original suffering you were trying to avoid by engaging in eating disorder behaviors, recovery begins. If you are in this place, or if you have been working to find other ways to tolerate suffering, bring compassion, and engage in change, that is the place of recovery!

Feeling out of control, I would venture to say, happens for most mothers. But for us moms who have a predisposition to being extra sensitive to feeling out of control (and not liking it), it can be especially uncomfortable. The temptation might be to restrict, binge, or purge food in response to feeling out of control. And there's nothing like watching your body get larger and larger and larger, more and more pregnant, or trying to soothe a colicky newborn to trigger feeling out of control! If you're *not* engaging in eating disorder behaviors, guess what often emerges? Well, one possibility is anxiety. I see this frequently in clients with whom I work. When they stop engaging in behaviors, they report feeling more anxious. And guess what anxious women do when they are pregnant? Or postpartum? Worry. They worry about everything. They worry about labor and delivery.

They worry about preparing and (trying to) control everything. This is not all bad. As Pam England writes, "Worry is the work of pregnancy... an overconfident first-time mom who thinks she has it all figured out, worries me. I worry she will not be truly prepared for what awaits her." Some common worries she mentions include: not being able to stand the pain, not being able to relax, feeling rushed, or fear of taking too long, pelvis not being big enough, cervix not opening, lack of privacy, being judged for making noise, being separated from the baby, having to fight for or request to be respected, having an intervention that is not necessary.[99]

As "worry is the work of pregnancy," this worry is not necessarily all counterproductive. When I used to work at a residential treatment program for women recovering from eating disorders, I would praise the clients who were afraid – and worried – as they prepared to discharge from treatment. If they weren't worried about their recovery, I was! If they were scared, they knew that they needed to be mindful about protecting their recovery. Recovery takes attention and vigilance to protect. Overconfidence can invite failure or relapse. It's all about the right balance. Too much worry can be debilitating. Not enough worry can invite harm.

Be vigilant about your eating disorder and/or mood disorder recovery and invite support. If you are struggling with anxiety or depression, or relapsing into your eating disorder, get support. One important factor to know is that there is a difference between worrying about labor and delivery and a full-blown mood disorder. If you are not sleeping, if you are having intrusive thoughts or panic attacks, if you are feeling constantly irritable, hypervigilant, anger bordering on rage, or constantly weepy, these are signs of a mood disorder. These are not the only signs. Mood disorders can show up in many different forms. Talk to a professional who specializes in perinatal mood disorders. Talk therapy and medication can and have both been shown to be effective in recovery. The sooner you get support in place, the better.

Pregnancy has been recognized as a time when women may be particularly motivated for eating disorder recovery, so it is a good time to set up support for yourself. (For example, you may have more energy and ability to attend therapy appointments in person when you are pregnant than postpartum.) However, *it is never a bad time to reach out for support.* And many therapists and psychiatrists who specialize in perinatal care have flexibility with bringing your baby to appointments or offering telemedicine where it is appropriate.

After the Birth

If you are making a birth plan, make sure to include what happens afterward. This is where it is so important to make sure you have support in place. Have your partner, mom, doulas, support group, therapist, perinatal psychiatrist (or preferably some combination of or all of the above) on deck. Try not to wait until after the birth to set this up. Remember: *postpartum is the highest risk time for relapse in your eating disorder, and for a perinatal mood disorder.*

What are some ways to prepare for postpartum? I went back to Britt Forman, the doula, to ask how she supports new moms postpartum, and here is what she said:

> Support entails getting prepared ahead of time. In the prenatal visits we're talking about who they imagine having around them, what resources they have available to them, and whether their plan is realistic. If they say, "My mother-in-law is going to come for the first two weeks," I ask, "How do you get along with your mother-in-law?"
>
> If the answer is, "Not very well. I'll probably have to take care of her along with the baby," then that's not a realistic plan.
>
> I strongly encourage them to plan for a minimum of two weeks of staying in bed postpartum. This helps their physical body

recover from the birth, helps facilitate skin-to-skin contact and bonding with the baby, and reduces strain on their pelvic floor. I encourage them to sleep as much as possible, even if it's only in small increments.

In our postpartum visit, I'm making sure the plan they had set in place is actually working. If it seems like they need more resources, then I will help them connect with postpartum doulas, lactation consultants, body workers, meal delivery, or other resources, so that they can get what they need.

I'm also available for processing whatever is coming up for them. I find that women often need someone besides their partner that they can talk to about what is coming up for them. For a lot of women with their first babies [especially if they are accomplished career women, recovering from an eating disorder, or both], this is unlike any experience they've ever had before. It can be really hard emotionally to feel like all they're doing is lying around feeding a baby. They feel like they "should" be doing more. Or doing a "better" job than they're doing, even when things are going well. It's such unknown terrain. It's a completely foreign experience.

Birth [labor and delivery] is unknown and foreign, but that is finite. In postpartum, the altered state wears off, and new moms can feel exhausted and depleted. They may feel trapped under the weight of new motherhood. I get to be someone to normalize the feelings. New moms can be isolated and get sucked into a black hole of feelings. If we just have someone to hold space for us, we can let some of the heaviness go and have a better perspective: this is a big transition! And these feelings are temporary – just like the feelings of labor were temporary.

A Note about Food

I'm not going to get specific about food, in order not to be triggering. But here is what I will say: you probably need to eat more than you think you need to postpartum. Here's what Britt had to say about food and eating:

> The way that women are nourished with their food, postpartum, is really important. They need nutrient-dense food. They need to have support in place to be eating on a 24-hour clock, not just three meals a day, like they're used to. Their partner can support them in the rhythm of feeding, by feeding Mom when they feed the baby. [This is an opportunity for you to receive, Mom. I know it's hard. Try to say yes.] Postpartum women need to have food at the ready: by their bedside, next to the toilet, next to the rocking chair, or wherever they are hanging out, so they can easily snack throughout the 24 hours a day. Staying truly and deeply nourished is part of maintaining wellness, healthy brain chemistry, maintaining milk supply, and supporting postpartum healing.

Postpartum Supplies

Here are a couple more pragmatic tips. Have extra-absorbent menstrual pads at hand. You may want to put them in a Ziploc bag and freeze them. Then you can take them out as needed, and they may feel soothing when cold. Some doulas add aloe or herbs to these "padsicles."[100]

If you had a C-section, you may want pain medication. Talk with your doctor about appropriate treatment, and whether the medication is safe if you are going to be breastfeeding.

Make food ahead of time and freeze it so you will have meals. I love this saying I heard from Monique the doula: "Fed is best."[101] Just as it is important to make sure you are feeding your new baby (and breast isn't always best, but *fed* is), it is important you are feeding you! Don't forget to eat.

If the voice of your eating disorder says:

You're just lying in bed. You don't need to eat,

tell it:

F* off. When you grow a human and give birth to it, you can offer your opinion. Until then, you are not in charge of the decision making. (And even then, I'm not taking visitors like you.)

After giving birth you need to rest, hydrate, and eat. In some cultures, this is the custom for 40 days after giving birth. The first 40 days after the birth of a baby offer an important period of rest and recovery for new mothers. Heng Ou writes of her postpartum experience with *zuo yuezi*, a set period of "confinement," in which a woman remains at home and eats food (no cold food, special postpartum soups) prepared by relatives, who move in to assist in caring for her during this time.[102]

Some Latina women practice *cuarentena*, which is a postpartum period during which the new mom abstains from sex and focuses only on breastfeeding and taking care of her baby and herself. Other family members cook and clean for her and the baby during these 40 days.[103]

You may not be able to, or want to, have relatives come stay with you for 40 days postpartum. However, if friends or family members offer to make you a meal, say yes. You are welcome to take the meal, but not invite them to visit. Tell them you're not ready. Or have your partner/ spouse say, "You need to leave now – she needs rest." If the person is a good friend, they will understand. Also, hydrate. Make sure to drink water! Frequently!

In Conclusion

The right kind of support is important. When the right kind of sup...
offered, accept the support. If your friend, mom, dad, or mother-in-law is
intrusive and offers unsolicited advice or non-stop (uninteresting) gossip,
set a boundary. You can do this kindly, but do it. You are the mom now, so
you get to decide. If you don't want visitors, or you don't want visitors for
more than 15 minutes, say it. Or have your spouse/partner say it.

Do let yourself be supported, though. There is a difference between
restorative time and isolation. This can be tricky to differentiate. I remember
not wanting anyone to see me postpartum when I was in the third-day-
wearing-the-same-sweatpants. Your partner, true friends, relatives, and
especially fellow moms will understand the postpartum-sweatpants stage.
That's not a good reason to decline support. That's isolating. A good reason
to decline support (visitors) is if you need rest. Feeling like you look "ugly
and disgusting" (yes, I know those are not feelings) in sweatpants is not.
Here is what Crystal, mama of five(!), has to say, which I could not have
said better:

> Recovery, like mothering, is not a process to be perfected. It is a
> journey of learning to adapt to disciplines of love for yourself and
> your body: in how you eat, in how you rest, in your thoughts, words,
> and actions. It is caring for yourself in the same way that you mother
> and care for your own children, with great love. Love is action and
> taking steps of daily faith, regardless of feeling or circumstance.
>
> If you are a mother in eating disorder recovery, you deserve
> compassionate encouragement, each and every step of the way.
>
> Through any doubts, insecurities or challenges that you might
> encounter on your motherhood journey, never stop believing that
> you are worthy, that you are deserving of compassion and self-
> respect. Regardless of your past, you were chosen to mother your
> children and are the best mama for them.

6
Good Breast, Bad Breast, Good Enough Breast

—— ♡ ——

It's Not "Breast Is Best"; It's Fed Is Best – Stop "Shoulding" on Yourself and Find the Right Answer for You

Breastfeeding was quite the experience for the first few months. Tongue clipped twice,[104] pumping challenges, finger feeder... It didn't look anything like those posters that are plastered all over the lactation consultants' offices... You know the ones, where the baby is lovingly looking into the mom's eyes and the mom is looking lovingly at baby, smiling brightly, while hair and makeup look fabulous... Yeah, pretty much the opposite.

– First-time mom

Breastfeeding is hard. As a card sent to me in early motherhood by a friend stated:

Whoever said, "There's no use crying over spilled milk" never pumped 6 ounces of it out of their breast and then accidentally knocked it over.

The image of the glowing mother feeding the perfectly latched-on baby suckling with euphoria rarely matches up with reality. One UC Davis

Medical Center study found that 92 percent of the new moms they surveyed reported at least one breastfeeding concern three days after birth.[105] Breastfeeding problems are extremely common and increase the possibility of abandoning breastfeeding altogether.

Here is a list of possible challenges that can come with breastfeeding: breast engorgement, plugged milk duct, breast infection, insufficient milk supply, thrush, breast pain, mastitis, sore nipples, nipple confusion, cracked or bleeding nipples, tongue tie or other oral anatomy issues, overactive letdown and/or fast flow, slow infant weight gain, feeding with a history of breast surgery, feeding a preterm baby, breast anatomy (inverted, flat, or large nipples), sleepy babies, breast refusal.

Breast Is Not Always Best

Most of us, before becoming moms, had no idea. I remember sitting in a breastfeeding preparation class with other pregnant moms and partners. I innocently raised my hand and asked about formula feeding. I thought I would try breastfeeding, and if it didn't work for me, then I'd switch to formula. For a moment, when the room went silent, I was confused then felt the quiet shame. Oh, I realized, you're not supposed to ask that question.

But for many women, breastfeeding is not the best option. Moms who are survivors of sexual abuse can be triggered in many ways during the experience of breastfeeding. Breast exposure, secretions, sensations from suckling or stroking, and continuous demands from the baby can feel too overwhelming.[106]

Penny Simpkin, a doula, childbirth educator, and counselor, has articulated many of the issues that can arise for these moms, including modesty around exposing their breasts, feelings of disgust, pain, or flashbacks to abuse brought on by baby having access to breasts. She makes suggestions for lactation consultants working with these moms such as acknowledging that sometimes abuse survivors cannot breastfeed and pumping or feeding by bottle may work better. She also suggests teaching latch techniques that allow for privacy, not touching a woman's breasts, and helping these moms recognize that young babies (unlike adult abusers) cannot *deliberately* hurt or manipulate her. For these moms especially, maintaining a sense of their own control, choices, and autonomy is important for them to feel empowered and at ease.

For many moms, not just survivors of abuse, having a lactation consultant or nurse touch, grab, or manipulate their breasts can feel uncomfortable. A breastfeeding friend of mine referred to lactation consultants as "the Breast Generals." I remember sitting in a new-mom group myself, thinking, *"What if I wasn't breastfeeding? Where would I get support?"* So many new-moms' groups are led by lactation consultants who (understandably) hold the belief that Breast Is Best.

It is OK to choose not to breastfeed!

The Virgin–Whore Dichotomy

Many women do not feel comfortable breastfeeding in public or exposing their breasts, even if they don't have a history of abuse. I remember one moment when my husband and I were at a restaurant, and the waiter came to take our beverage orders. I was breastfeeding our baby, and while my husband and I were giving our orders I could feel the waiter looking at my breast. I looked the waiter in the eye and said, "He's all set."

Everybody laughed. It was my joking but fierce way of saying, "Stop looking at my breast!"

Contrary to my former, pre-baby self, who felt anticipatory anxiety about breastfeeding in public, my post-baby self actually didn't care. I was too f*ing tired. Also, the baby wouldn't feed under a "hooter hider." (Yes, they really are called that – those cloth scarves that hang over your breast and baby while feeding. I'm not sure who, exactly, they thought they were marketing to. Most moms I know do not refer to their breasts as "hooters.")

I did experience the strange double standard that American culture holds around women and breasts. Women's breasts are displayed all over media screens – in movies, magazines, porn, and in plastic surgery advertisements. But then, when a woman tries to breastfeed on an airplane, she is called "disgusting," and asked to cover up.[107]

I love this quote from the journalist Anna Quindlen:

> When an actress takes off her clothes onscreen, but a nursing mother is told to leave, what message do we send about the roles of women? In some ways we're as committed to the old Madonna-whore dichotomy as ever. And the Madonna stays home, feeding the baby behind the blinds, a vestige of those days when for a lady to venture out was a flagrant act of public exposure.[108]

If you are struggling with breastfeeding in public, you are not alone. The good news is that moms are a fierce tribe who look out for each other. When one mother was forced to check her breast pump as baggage in the airport, she started a Facebook group for breastfeeding moms who travel. It gained over 1000 followers in its first month.[109] As a result of social media pressure from breastfeeding moms, many airlines have been forced to improve policies and create rules that are: "not left to interpretation by an airline employee, and in turn harass/shame/bully a mother."[110]

What if I'm Taking Medication?

Moms who are on medication, psychiatric or otherwise, are often concerned about how it could affect their baby. According to the Centers for Disease Control:

Although many medications do pass into breast milk, most have no effect on milk supply or on infant well-being. Few medications are contraindicated while breastfeeding... A 2013 clinical report by the American Academy of Pediatrics (AAP) indicates that most medications and immunizations are safe to use during lactation.[111]

If you are on medication, or considering being on medication, you will need to check with your care provider, preferably a perinatal mood specialist, to see what the risks are with different medications. If you are considering psychiatric medication (which, along with therapy, is often the best treatment for perinatal mood disorders), you will need to assess, with your doctor, risks versus benefits, for both you and your baby. According to the American Academy of Pediatrics, healthcare providers should weigh the risks and benefits when prescribing medications to breastfeeding mothers by considering the many factors, including need for the medication by the mother, potential effects on breast milk production, the amount of the medication excreted into breast milk, potential adverse effects on the breastfeeding infant, and other factors.[112]

I do have a bias in encouraging you to please make sure to remember that *you* and your health are the most important factors to consider if you are recovering from anxiety, depression, or another mood disorder. If you are not well, your baby will suffer. I say this because shame can be both a symptom of a mood disorder (enhanced feelings of guilt about being a "bad mom") and a deterrent to getting treatment. The most important factor in treating postpartum depression is getting Mom back to health. As one extensive article on PPD points out:

It can be argued that the risks of exposure to PPD outweigh at least the short-term risks of infant exposure to antidepressants through breast milk, because the multiple negative effects of untreated PPD on short-term and long-term child development are well-established; in addition to the multiple known benefits for infants with breastfeeding.[113]

Do not let fear of being a bad mom stop you from getting treatment! And please remember that good (enough) moms choose to breastfeed, good (enough) moms choose to partially breastfeed, and good (enough) moms choose not to breastfeed.

A Word about Mommy Brain

I distinctly remember one moment, postpartum, when my husband and I were in a bookstore, with baby in the carrier, browsing. I saw the book *The Female Brain* and picked it up, thumbing directly to the section on "Mommy Brain," and, more specifically, "Breast Feeding and the Fuzzy Brain." I was still breastfeeding, fuzzy-brained, and seeking some scientific proof that I wasn't going crazy. I found it. Louann Brizendine, MD writes:

> one down side of breast feeding can be a lack of mental focus. Although a fuzzy brained state is pretty common after giving birth, breast feeding can heighten and prolong this mellow…unfocused state…the parts of the brain responsible for focus and concentration are preoccupied with protecting and tracking the newborn.[114]

If you are struggling with feeling like you lost your brain when you gave birth to your baby, don't worry. You are not alone, and it will come back. Although your brain, like your body, like you, will most likely be forever changed by becoming a mother.

Benefits of the Breast

Now that we have addressed some of the obstacles to breastfeeding, and some of the reasons women may choose not to do it, let's look at some of the benefits. For this chapter, I interviewed Jennifer Suffin, IBCLC. Jennifer is a perinatal educator and mother of two, who feels lucky to get to do what she loves and honored to share her knowledge and compassion with all different types of families, who may be feeding in any number of ways. She takes pride in offering her clients a sense of comfort and valuable, evidence-based tools to help empower them through (breast) feeding challenges and beyond.

Here is our Q & A:

What led you to the work of becoming a lactation consultant?

Becoming a mom was harder than I could have imagined. I knew I needed some sort of support, so I sought out my local new-mom support group. I had never considered myself a joiner, but finding this room of women and their little ones was the lifeline I needed to help make those early months more manageable and enjoyable. I, of course, learned from those in attendance, and, subsequently, in my work, that the challenges I was facing (in my case: intense anxiety and a sense of loss of self) were not unique. It made all the difference in the world to have this proverbial "village" to count on to help me understand my feelings and the logistics of caring for a newborn that many of us are unaware of in our culture, due to living so far from our families. I gained some confidence through the support of these women, and when my best friend suggested I should become a lactation consultant, after helping her get through her initial challenges with her newborn, I was intrigued and excited. I began my studies shortly thereafter and haven't looked back since. I absolutely love my work, which I have been lucky enough to do for the last ten years.

What are some of the benefits of breastfeeding?

Breast milk provides optimal levels of vitamins and nutrients for your specific baby. It is easily digestible. It provides antibodies against illness and infection, and it lowers the risk of asthma, allergies, infections, and diarrhea.

Some studies have shown that breastfeeding is linked to higher IQ scores later in life. The act of breastfeeding itself, as you would imagine, promotes bonding and a sense of security through eye contact, physical closeness, and skin-to-skin touching. Breastfeeding plays a role in learning satiety cues, which can reduce the risk of weight issues in the future. The American Academy of Pediatrics has come out, saying that breastfeeding plays a role in the prevention of SIDS (sudden infant death syndrome). Although more research is needed, breastfeeding has been thought to lower the risk of diabetes and certain cancers.

Are there breastfeeding benefits for the mother?

Breastfeeding is potentially protective against postpartum depression, due to the hormones released during feeding. These hormones are released in response to suckling and cuddling. One specific hormone, oxytocin, which is one of your "feel good" hormones, helps your uterus return to its pre-pregnancy size and may reduce uterine bleeding after birth. Breastfeeding burns extra calories, so for some, it can help them lose their pregnancy weight faster. Breastfeeding also lowers your risk of breast and ovarian cancer, and there are some studies that show it may lower your risk of osteoporosis.

What comes up for, and what are some of the ways you work with, women in their breastfeeding/new-mom struggles?

Going back to the notion that we often live so isolated from our families and loved ones in these times, moms are often stunned at how challenging having a new baby can be, because they have not vicariously experienced what it is like to care for and spend time with a newborn. I would have to say that the overriding theme I most often encounter is moms feeling so surprised at how hard breastfeeding can be for some, despite the fact that it is "supposed to just work and be natural" (as we have done for millennia). Also, because new moms don't have many longer-term examples to look to, it is often difficult for moms to see that things will constantly be changing, often for the better. What we experience in the first week of life will be quite different from what we experience in the third month of life, but moms are unable to picture what that might look like when they are in the thick of trying to get their baby to gain the weight they may have lost after birth, all while on four hours of sleep in the last 24.

My goal for any new family I work with is to offer warm support, gentle encouragement, and a true sense of empowerment, while providing practical, evidence-based tools to guide them in their individual experience.

How do you help new moms with body shame (postpartum body-image distress; breasts not making enough milk; women for whom anxiety is triggered in their bodies because of a history of abuse)?

I make sure I am fully present, and I listen. My practice is structured so I can spend a good amount of time listening to a mom's story. One of my mentors once told me that lactation consulting is 10 percent clinical, 90 percent counseling. My undergraduate background is in psychology, so I have a definite interest in helping moms understand why they are feeling what they are feeling, validating those feelings, and then helping them to come up with ways to look at things from a different perspective. Breastfeeding is such an intimate act, and as such, it can bring about a tremendous shift in a woman's understanding of herself. It can touch on challenging notes in her history or put a spotlight on the expectations she has for herself. My role is often to normalize some of these types of feelings, make sure the mom feels heard, and to never push or pressure any agenda. I meet moms, within the family dynamic, where they are, and structure a plan that feels manageable and progressive. I stay in touch for some time after the in-person visit, not only to be able to support the plan we established together, but to continue to offer encouragement and understanding. I often refer my clients to other trusted practitioners such as psychologists and sleep consultants, based on the things they share with me. I value the relationships I have with other practitioners and find that moms getting this kind of comprehensive care often fare better as they move forward.

What about the mother guilt that can come with choosing to supplement breast milk with formula, being on medication for perinatal mood and anxiety disorders, or choosing to stop breastfeeding?

Mother guilt is huge, especially in this age of prevalent social media. We often see others' "perfect" lives and have difficulty teasing out what is likely the truth. Rather, we compare our un-showered selves to the improbable. When mother guilt comes up, I try to encourage moms to recognize that by making the choices that feel right for them, they are actually tapping into what really makes them a good mother. We can't be all things, all the time, to our children. We need to replenish ourselves, and by doing so, we come back to our children with renewed energy and purpose, and our children ultimately benefit.

I would add that it is super-important to find your "village." If we can't live near our families (and some of us don't want to), we need to create our own. When new moms are ready, joining a support group in person is ideal, but even those online can provide the connection and understanding that we are not alone in our challenges and triumphs. Together we are stronger. This goes a long way during those early days of awe, and beyond.

Jennifer's advice mirrors that of a guide to new moms and breastfeeding, and recommends the following:

- Expect the unexpected. There may (or may not) be problems at first, or later on.
- Line up a an International Board Certified Lactation Consultant, even before the baby comes. (Jennifer stresses this credential is important, as the IBCLC credential is much more rigorous and thorough than other trainings. In addition, many people can call themselves a "lactation specialist" with little or no training, experience, or mentoring.)
- Don't sweat a little supplementation with formula.
- Create your own support network for breastfeeding.[115]

This last point – support – is an area that moms in other areas of the world have down. Himba moms in Namibia, for instance, often live with their mothers after giving birth, and the mother mentors the new mom on breastfeeding. Brooke Scelza, an evolutionary anthropologist at the University of Los Angeles, California, hypothesized that long, uninterrupted contact after birth helps support the newborn's suckling instinct. Another cultural factor is that Himba women learn how to breastfeed throughout their childhood, by seeing their moms, siblings, and friends breastfeed while growing up.[116]

Good Breasts, Bad Breasts, Good Enough Breasts

I'm going to put on my psychologist hat for just a moment to look at being a good (enough) mom to yourself in order to be a good (enough) mom to your baby. Bear with me as I take a mini, tangential-but-relevant journey into psychological theory.

Melanie Klein, one of the founders of a school of thought called "object relations," which grew out of Freud's psychodynamic theory, coined the term "good breast, bad breast."[117] This concept refers to the idea that infants "split" the experience of their mothers into "bad" (frustrating, hated) and "good" (loving, gratifying) objects. This "splitting," she postulates, is essential for the infant to take in and hold onto a good experience and keep at bay the overwhelming bad experience. Establishing this "goodness" inside helps the infant (child, adult) work through feelings of guilt or grief over hating the "bad breast" part of the mother.[118]

For women recovering from eating disorders, there is often a deeply held belief about being "bad" or "not good enough." For many different reasons, depending on our own early attachment with caregivers, temperament, and traumatic life experiences, we often feel we are "bad" (flawed, inadequate). So, when we become mothers ourselves, this cultural ideal around motherhood – how you should be glowing, breastfeed perfectly and easily, never feel inadequate or unfulfilled – contrasts especially starkly with our actual experience. And we think, because we're not having this "perfect" motherhood experience, we are bad, flawed, not good enough.

If you feel this way, I want to encourage you to keep coming back to mothering *yourself* differently, along with learning how to mother your little one. When you have a feeling of inadequacy, try, to the best of your ability, to take a deep breath and tell yourself you are good enough. Try to imagine all the other mothers in this messy soup of new parenthood. Imagine a dear friend of yours having the same struggle as you, and the kindness and cheerleading you would offer them.

There is no "right," perfect-for-everyone answer. There is the good enough answer for you and your family, right now. Some moms breastfeed well into their child's toddler years; some moms never breastfeed; most moms fall into the large spectrum of possibilities between these two choices. All moms have the opportunity to practice being "good enough." So, when your overdeveloped mama critic starts telling you that you are a bad mom, please tell it:

Thank you for sharing. We are now ready to hear any further opinions from the voice of a friend.

The Good Enough, Imperfect Mother

The term "good enough mother" was first coined by Donald Winnicott, a British psychoanalyst and pediatrician. Winnicott, after observing thousands of babies and their mothers, realized that children actually benefit from their mothers failing them (in small, daily ways, not from abuse or neglect). When our babies are newborns, we tend to their needs almost immediately, whether it be feeding, diapering, or soothing. As they grow, we still try to do this. But, inevitably, we fail them by not being able to meet their needs immediately, or by responding imperfectly. This prepares them to live in an imperfect world and tolerate the distress of that world.[119] To be clear, I'm not talking about abuse or neglect. I'm talking about how when your little one falls off their bike for the first time, it's going to hurt. You can't bubble wrap them to prevent this. (Believe me: if I could, I would have tried.)

Nutrition and Breastfeeding

My nutritionist colleagues want me to remind you: if you are breastfeeding, you need to eat more food and drink more water. I'm deliberately leaving out calorie count, to not be triggering. But you need more food. Your body will tell you, through its hunger and satiety cues, how much. Trust that.

It is especially important that you not engage in any restrictive eating or dieting during this time. And, in case you are not breastfeeding, and the voice of your eating disorder just said, *"Well, I'm not breastfeeding, so I can restrict,"* the answer is still a resounding *No.* That ship has sailed for you. Once you are in recovery, you know – no matter how much you may not want to acknowledge it – that diets don't work. Diets do not work, restricting makes you crazy, and the Fourth Law of Physics says that *every diet has an equal and opposite binge.*

I borrowed that last law of physics from Geneen Roth, a well-known author and advocate for disordered eating recovery. She advises eating what your body wants, with pleasure, enjoyment, and without distraction. She encourages us to pay attention to when we are hungry and when we have had enough, because "obsession and awareness cannot coexist."[120] I would also suggest that, since it is often *quite challenging* as a mom to eat without distraction, you practice taking one bite without distraction. Or perhaps, sitting down. How many of us moms are jiggling, juggling, and feeding the baby while eating at the same time? It happens. But try to sit down for one bite of your meal. And make sure you get a meal. You are not only worth it and good enough, you need it. You need food, and you need to take care of you.

In Conclusion

Wherever you are on your breastfeeding, not breastfeeding, breastfeeding with supplementing, considering throwing your breast pump out the window trajectory, please practice being a good mom to yourself, knowing you are doing the best you can. And please get support. Remember: you are good enough.

7
Distress Tolerance

——— ♡ ———

How to Successfully Not Be Supermom
(and Be OK with It)

When my mom was mothering, the general consensus was: if you feed your kids,
you're doing great. Just ring a cowbell when it is time for them to come home for
(canned green beans and non-organic mac and cheese casserole) dinner.

Today, we're supposed to pre-screen all food for BPA-free packaging or
home-make baby food with all organic ingredients. We're supposed to sing
classical music to our babies and get them on the waiting list for preschool
– and the right Ivy League college – while we are still pregnant. We're
supposed to show Baby Einstein videos, but share absolutely no screens
before preschool. Please try and find me a mom who has been able to keep
her phone out of the hands of her toddler.

– Mom, 2018

When I was in Postpartum Support International's perinatal mood
disorders training, Wendy Davis, PhD, discussed the theory of how
temperament factors can play a role in predisposing certain women
to postpartum depression or anxiety.[121] A few of the main ones were
perfectionism, overachieving, and self-reliance. Women with these
perfectionistic temperaments were most likely to try to be "Supermom,"

and therefore have more distress around the massive learning curve of new motherhood. *"Aha!"* I thought, *"That makes so much sense!"* Given the "risk aversion" and "high sensitivity to rejection and failure" temperaments of most women recovering from eating disorders, these women, in particular, are set up to have a rough journey with new motherhood.[122]

Risk aversion, just like it sounds, is the tendency to avoid taking risks. Dr. Craig Johnson, a psychologist and eating disorder specialist, refers to people with this tendency as "turtles." Turtles, when faced with risk, hide or avoid. They pull back from, instead of going toward, scary, new situations. Well, pregnancy and new motherhood are *full* of scary, new situations! Given the current cultural context of most new parents – not living in a community where they have been surrounded by infants (and their new parents) being cared for by a whole village – new parenthood is full of the scariness of the new. In today's Western culture, most first-time moms have never been to an actual birth, seen or assisted with a new mom breastfeeding, changed a diaper, or attempted to soothe a colicky baby. All of these realities can come as quite a shock if the only context a woman has had access to prior to actual motherhood was Hollywood's place-a-fake-bump-under-the-actress's-shirt, have-a-five-minute-labor-and-delivery, and live-happily-ever-after version. As you've just read, or are currently experiencing, the contrasting reality of attempting breastfeeding alone can overwhelm even the most competent of new moms.

I know no one told me how difficult it can be to breastfeed. I thought, prior to becoming a mom, you just pop that baby on your boob, and that's it! And how hard can it be to take a shower? Those new moms who struggle with that must just be lazy, I thought. After having my baby, I remember talking with a further-along-mom, a super-accomplished therapist, musician, and dressage teacher, about how humbling new mommy-hood was. She shared with me how her goal, for a day, in the early postpartum period was to get a load of laundry in the washer. That's it. And she didn't even try to take a shower. Just get one load of laundry into the washer. That was a good day.

A mantra another recovery mama and I continue to repeat to each other, even now, with our children being four, five, and six years old, is: *lower the bar*. Whatever your expectation is: lower the bar. New motherhood, like new recovery, requires throwing perfectionism out the window. It also calls on the recovery skill of not "comparing and despairing."

Some Thoughts about "Compare and Despair"

Women recovering from eating disorders *love* to "compare and despair." They see another mom who they determine to be better than them in some way, and then despair at their own inadequacy. Usually there is not much evidence gathered to determine how these other moms are better. Often these "perfect" moms are found on social media. I hear countless versions of "the perfect mother" in weekly therapy sessions with my clients. When I ask where these perfect mothers are, I am often told they are found on: Instagram, Facebook, or Pinterest.

"So, these aren't real mothers," I say.

"Yes, they are!" my clients protest.

"Have you sat in on their therapy session this week?"

"Well, nooooo…"

Did you see the photo – that they didn't post – of their child having a green food-spewing tantrum right after the photo of them happily spooning the organic homemade spinach into the child's mouth? Or the one of them in their bathing suit – before it was edited? Or did you listen in on the fight they had with their partner about who was going to do the laundry this week, after they took that smiling photo of the family hiking together?

If you are going to compare and despair, be fair. Here is a body-image example. If you are struggling with getting into a bathing suit postpartum, while looking at celebrities, six weeks after birth, in their bikinis (*personal trainer, personal chef, full-time nanny and night doula assisted, followed by mommy tuck and airbrushing on the photos*), that's not fair. If you are going to compare yourself, then go to a mommy-and-me swim class with other moms and babes and see if they look like those cellulite-free celebrities.

Oh, and while you are there with the real moms, strike up a conversation. One of them might become a good friend, in Real Life!

Support

Support can be tricky as a new mom. If you're a person who shies away from new experiences or waits to be seen until you have mastered a skill, then you are likely to be a mom who isolates (and is at risk for depression, anxiety, or eating disorder relapse). But support is crucial to challenging perfectionistic versions of unrealistic motherhood.

When I was a new mom, I went to a new-moms' group where we were all struggling along with breastfeeding, being bored, worrying about our baby's poop and our postpartum bodies. I won't say it was fun, but there was an element of what Dr. Kristin Neff, who introduced the practice of mindful self-compassion, calls "common humanity." The Wall Street moms, the doctor moms, the stay-at-home moms, the teacher moms, the advanced-maternal-age and the twenty-something moms were all sitting at the same table. Motherhood is what some call "the great leveler." We were all in it together, and each of us had as much experience and as few answers as the rest of us. Although I still struggled with feelings of isolation and not belonging, this helped. It helped to know I was not alone.

I'm not going to idealize "the olden days" here, but I will say that there has been a cultural trend away from connection with extended family. There is more value being placed on trying to do new parenthood alone than there used to be. This can be painful. Professional supports such as doulas, lactation consultants, and therapists can help. But these resources are not financially available to everyone.

If you are reading this and feeling alone, know that you are not. Just take a moment and take a deep breath. Breathe in all the moms who have gone before you and struggled with the very same experiences you are going through. Whether it be struggling with food and body image, being unable to breastfeed, being up every night at 3 a.m., being bone-weary exhausted, being bored, alone all day for eight hours with an infant, or struggling with depression or anxiety, there have been many other moms who have traveled this very road you are on. (I also want you to get in-person support, especially if you are struggling with an eating or perinatal mood disorder. See the Resources section at the end of the book to find resources for support.) For this breath, may you know that you are not alone. With 7.5 billion people on this planet, know that another person has had, or is having, right at the same time with you, this experience. And they survived or are surviving. And they thrived; or they struggled at first, and now they are thriving.

This is the spiritual practice aspect of breaking isolation (more on this in Chapter 8). Breathe in kindness for you and every other mother who is going through what you are going through. Imagine and see them in your mind's eye. Send them this awareness you are having right now: of not being alone, of allowing imperfection, of temporarily stopping the comparing and despairing, the isolation, and the fear that this will never get better. It will. You will get through this. You *are* getting through this.

Radical Acceptance

You may be asking *but how?* This is where skills like "radical acceptance" come in. Radical acceptance is one of the skills in DBT. Marsha Linehan is the founder of DBT, which, as it sounds, works with dialectics.[123] In other words, it allows you both to like and hate being a mom. It allows you to be struggling and be at peace with the struggle, at the same time. It allows you to want to change, to be changing, and to be accepting of exactly where you are.

Mindfulness teacher Tara Brach has this to say:

> We suffer because we have forgotten who we are, and our identity has become confined to the sense of a separate, usually deficient self. All difficult emotions – fear and anger, shame and depression – arise out of this trance of what I call false self... I've found that whenever I am really suffering, on some level I am believing and feeling that "something is wrong with me."[124]

Inside distressing feelings, inside depression, inside the immense rite of passage that is motherhood, *there is nothing wrong with you.* You don't always have to like the experience of motherhood. Tara states:

> Radical acceptance has two elements: it is an honest acknowledgment of what is going on inside you, and a courageous willingness to be with life in the present moment, just as it is. I sometimes simplify it to "recognizing" and "allowing..." You can accept an experience without liking it.[125]

You may be thinking, but how can I accept what I don't like? You may say, as my clients frequently do, "You want me to just 'sit with this'?" Well, yes, and no. Part of radical acceptance does include "sitting with" the experience, even if you don't like it. And you can also use other skills to help tolerate the distress and create change.

What Is Distress Tolerance?

If you've given birth, no matter what your birth story is, you have experienced distress. All labor and deliveries are distressing. You have tolerated it (or you will tolerate it), experienced (or will experience) it, and moved (or will travel) through it. Marsha Linehan coined the term "distress tolerance." She states:

> DBT emphasizes learning to bear pain skillfully. The ability to tolerate and accept distress is an essential mental health goal for at least two reasons. First, pain and distress are a part of life; they cannot be entirely avoided or removed. The inability to accept this immutable fact itself leads to increased pain and suffering. Second, distress tolerance, at least over the short run, is part and parcel of any attempt to change oneself; otherwise…actions will interfere with efforts to establish desired changes.[126]

Bearing pain skillfully means holding the awareness that "this is what it is" and "this will pass" simultaneously. It is a strange paradox that by accepting the pain of the moment, it often helps alleviate it.

A recovery friend of mine uses this literal metaphor. While driving in her car, she finds herself fiddling with the temperature controls, radio, and other dials. She is constantly trying to "get it right": not too cold, not too hot, just the right music, etc. But the more she fiddles, the more restless and irritable it tends to make her. Now, instead, she practices putting a song on the radio and listening to it, the whole way through. I'm not saying you should drive around in the freezing snow with no heat. What I am saying is distress tolerance involves a level of acceptance that, just because you don't like things the way they are, doesn't mean you have to change them in order to accept them.

Your baby is going to cry. You may have a colicky baby. Those of you who do know that you can try many, many things to stop this baby from crying, but some of them will work and *some of them will not*. And part of the experience of helping soothe the baby (*and yourself*) includes accepting that this is what it is. This experience, exactly as it is, is what you are going through right now. If you are someone who struggles with wanting to be "productive," or perhaps might be a tiny bit (or hugely, glaringly) perfectionistic, then you will have many opportunities to practice this distress tolerance skill while having a new baby and being a new mom. For example, let's say your baby is screaming, and you feel like screaming. Instead, you pause, take a deep breath, and say to yourself, *"Here we go. I have to deal with this right now. I don't like it, but it will pass."*

"Regulating Affect"

"Any successful therapy includes effectively learning to regulate affect."

I heard this sentence at a training workshop I was doing on trauma recently.[127] Rather than dismiss this as a bunch of clinical terminology mumbo jumbo, as I would in the past, this actually struck me as something to ponder deeply. First, I thought about this as it relates to myself and my clients. Regulating affect refers to the ability to moderate feelings skillfully. Whether it be bringing compassion to one's self, taking medication as prescribed for anxiety or depression, practicing challenging false assumptions around perfectionism or catastrophizing, or looking at ways in which you weren't met emotionally by your own parents and learning to meet yourself differently in the present – all of these interventions assist with regulating your emotions.

Then I thought about this idea as it relates to developing a close and secure relationship with a baby... Yep. Still applies. Babies need help with regulating their emotions! How do good moms do that? They hold them, rock them, soothe them, make shushing noises that resemble being in the womb, and either feed them (if it is physical hunger) or provide something else for them to suck on to self-soothe (if the hunger is more emotionally based).

Many of the adult clients I work with notice that the maladaptive behaviors that we work with alleviating (for example, bingeing, restricting or purging food) are attempts to regulate their emotions. Think about it: if you've ever eaten when you felt sad or angry, drank a glass of wine when you were feeling socially anxious, or gone shopping when feeling insecure or bored, you were most likely trying to change your feelings. You were trying to help regulate yourself. Even "process addictions," such as codependency, revolve around trying to soothe your own discomfort. Some of the ways I work with clients to understand how codependency can become addictive are by encouraging them to ask themselves: Do I need my partner to be OK for me to be OK? Do I take care of someone else at the expense of – or distraction from – myself? Do I take care of – or seek the company of – someone else in order to avoid or numb my own discomfort? Do I think I am the only person in the world who can help this (adult) person or that they are not capable of helping themselves?

There isn't actually anything wrong with these behaviors...until the pain caused by the behavior becomes greater than the original discomfort you were trying to avoid. This is the point where most people enter therapy.

I remember when I was a new mom and I would look forward to going to the coffee shop to get a treat when out with baby, strolling.

There wasn't anything wrong with this, until I realized one day that I was planning my day around getting to the coffee shop treat. This was a clue. "Loss of pleasure" is one of the key components in depression. I had literally lost any sense of pleasure, except for looking forward to this one moment in the day. It was time to increase the items in my toolbox, in terms of pleasurable activities, and widen my circle of support.

In Conclusion… Back to Compare and Despair

Here's what you can do when you find yourself isolating and comparing yourself to that Pinterest/Instagram/Facebook mom: imagine her in her therapy session. Imagine her talking about the same struggle you are going through. Imagine her struggling to live with a postpartum belly, find work–life balance, get enough sleep, not have time to make homemade, organic baby food. Imagine her feeling ambivalent about being a mom. Send her love. That's right: send the "perfect" mom love. Because you know who that perfect mom is? She's you. We have met the enemy, and she is us. Every mom struggles. This is part of the experience of humanity. Send her love and wish her well with finding the answer she needs, right now.

There is no perfect answer and there is no perfect mom. Take a deep breath into your postpartum belly and relax into the imperfection of right now. This is it. And it is (you are) enough.

8

Spirituality, Recovery, and Motherhood

——— ♡ ———

Finding Time to Meditate, Dance, Collage, Journal, Be Present, or Go to the Bathroom Alone, Even if It Is Five Minutes a Day

I was working full time, I was newly married, and life was taking on a new momentum. I had only really known yoga as a physical practice. Like I go someplace and I do yoga. I was running out of time to go to do yoga. Then I had my first child. And there was no yoga. There was no sleep, much less going to do yoga! There was nothing except full-time mom... Years later, I had my second daughter and it was at that point that I relapsed quite severely... As painful as that was, and as hard as that was, so many gifts that come from that relapse... That's when I learned that yoga is pausing to take a deep breath. That's when I learned the philosophies and all of the ways that we can live our lives as the practice of yoga. So now I don't have to go somewhere to do yoga... Can we breathe when we feel like we're going to explode? Can we keep ourselves grounded? How can we use yoga as a tool to help keep moving forward in our recovery?

– Jennifer Kreatsoulas, author, yoga therapist, and mother of two

When I first got into recovery for my eating disorder 20 years ago, I had three guidelines for spiritual practice:

1. Do it every day at the same time.
2. Do it, no matter what you are feeling.
3. Make it about the process, not the product.

This practice helped me dis-identify from the overly critical voice of the eating disorder and find a deeper place of knowing inside myself. It helped me find, and re-find, every day, the still, quiet voice of inner knowing. My spiritual practice changed throughout the years. For a long time, it consisted of writing in the morning and meditating every evening. Then it evolved into daily art/collage in my journal and movement as a meditation practice. Just like recovery, my spiritual practice had to evolve with me. Enter: pregnancy. Enter: the practice of morning sickness interferes with Morning Pages. Exit: Morning Pages and enter saltine crackers in bed prior to arising! This was the beginning of learning how to creatively fit spiritual practice in with the reality of becoming a mom. I had to start to learn the art of flow, of going with things in their natural rhythm, rather than directing and controlling things the way I wanted them to go: at the same time, predictably, every day.

A Word About "The G Word"

When I got into recovery, two decades ago, I was introduced to asking "God as you understand God" for help. For many recovering women, this concept can be triggering or feel like a minefield. Some women feel powerless in their eating disorder and want to find empowerment in themselves – not outside themselves – in their recovery. Some women, especially those who have a history of abuse from a man, feel uncomfortable giving their power to a masculine God, because a man who was in power used his power abusively toward them in the past. Other women find it redeeming to experience compassion and protection from a masculine God that they hadn't experienced previously. Stephanie Covington, author of *A Woman's Way Through the Twelve Steps*, writes:

> For many women, a discussion of spirit or spirituality throws us back into the religion of our childhood, an experience that we may feel very distant from or one that had no impact or a negative impact on our lives… For other women, religion has always been an important aspect of their lives and continues to shape their recovery process.[128]

In my early recovery experience, I found it important and empowering to discover the divine feminine. God was "Goddess" for me, for a long time. This helped me embrace having a feminine body, as well as other feminine aspects of myself that I had previously tried to cut myself off from in my eating disorder.

> Many women feel it is important to describe spiritual experience and their connection to the divine with female metaphors. For some women, spirituality is born from a profound sense of love for oneself that comes from a connection to the image of the goddess and the earth…the image of earth mother and earth goddess, depicted in fertility statues [with] rounded bellies and big and powerful breasts… Celebrating motherhood, birth, and creation puts us in touch with the power of the earth that creates and brings forth life.[129]

Later, during pregnancy, I embraced the Venus De Villendorf, an ancient feminine goddess of fertility, as a symbol of power and creation. This was particularly helpful when I struggled with the largeness (emotionally and bodily) of pregnancy and postpartum.

Many Names, No Name, Finding What Works for You

For some women, a connection with spirituality is connecting with "the part of you that knows." Andrea Wachter and Marsea Marcus, in their *Don't Diet, Live-It* workbook, write:

> We believe that within each of us exists a part that knows the truth – a part that knows when we just said "yes" and we really meant "no," a part that knows when we've had enough to eat or when we need more. Some call this their intuition. Some call it their gut, their heart, or their instinct. Some call it their Higher Power or God. We refer to it as "the part of you that knows."[130]

Marsha Linehan, the founder of DBT, calls this part of the self "Wise Mind." These words and concepts to identify parts of the self and spiritual experience are not completely overlapping. Each has its own distinct lineage. You can believe in more than one of these concepts, or just one of them, or have your own version that I have not named. You may believe in God and that God speaks to you through your Wise Mind. You may believe in the Great Mother Goddess and that she speaks to you through an intuitive part-of-you-that-knows. You may not believe in God/dess, but find solace, wisdom, and strength in an internal voice of compassionate knowing. Imaginal psychology calls this compassionately objective part of the self "the Friend." Carolyn Costin, a well-known eating disorder clinician, author, and international speaker, calls it "soul self."[131]

As I say to my recovering clients, there are many paths up the mountain. But it's the same mountain. You get to choose your path. The purpose of this chapter is not to tell you what the right spiritual path is for you. The point is to connect with your path. Whatever your concept of "the G word," and "the part of you that knows," it can be helpful to connect with this part in your recovery and motherhood journey. However, as a new mom, it can be challenging to find the time and quiet space for spiritual practice.

But I Don't Have Time to Pray and Meditate with a Newborn!

Denise Roy talks about Momfulness being "the spiritual practice of cultivating a mindful, compassionate, mothering presence." In her beautiful book, *Momfulness: Mothering with Mindfulness, Compassion, and Grace*, she writes:

> [In motherhood] Our perceptions about what constitutes spiritual practice may shift a bit. We might hold preconceived ideas about where to pray, how to meditate, what's supposed to happen, or what holiness looks like. In practicing Momfulness, we are much more likely to find ourselves meditating in a minivan than in a monastery! The delightful discovery we make, as we do these practices, is that there are innumerable sacred moments in our everyday family lives. We don't have to go anywhere else to find holy ground.[132]

In the beginning stages of postpartum, I stopped writing Morning Pages. If you haven't heard of Morning Pages, they are a form of "moving meditation" created by Julia Cameron, author of *The Artist's Way*, in which you free-write three pages every day, first thing upon arising:

> Morning Pages are three pages of longhand, stream of consciousness writing, done first thing in the morning. There is no wrong way to do Morning Pages – they are not high art. They are not even "writing." They are about anything and everything that crosses your mind – and they are for your eyes only. Morning Pages provoke, clarify, comfort,

cajole, prioritize and synchronize the day at hand. Do not over-think Morning Pages: just put three pages of anything on the page…and then do three more pages tomorrow.[133]

Sometimes I did afternoon pages. Sometimes I did Morning Pages in my mind. I would imagine draining my brain of any worries, anxieties, irritations, and fears onto the page. Though it didn't have the same effect (kind of like thinking about, rather than actually, meditating), it did help. It helped alleviate the constant worry and judgment that was going around and round in my sleep-deprived brain about how I "should" be doing more than I was. How had a whole day gone by, and all I had done was sat on the rug with baby and changed some diapers? Did I not used to be a *doctor* and a *contributing, intelligent member of society*? It was the ultimate spiritual practice of *don't just do something, sit there*: being bored on the floor with baby, feeling overwhelmed by diaper stink and laundry, getting all packed up ready to leave the house and having baby spew out a massive blow-out poop. I had to practice what Marsha Linehan calls radical acceptance.

What's Radical Acceptance? Radical means complete and total. It's when you accept something from the depths of your soul. When you accept it in your mind, in your heart, and even with your body. It's total and complete. When you've radically accepted something, you're not fighting it. It's when you stop fighting reality. That's what radical acceptance is.[134]

Like me, you might not be "a good floor mom." You can fight this, or you can accept it. I didn't like hanging out on the rug, jingling toys and building train tracks. However, when I accepted that, I was able to breathe deeply into the moment and glimpse a tiny bit of contentment and wonder.

In parenting, I have found what Jon Kabat-Zinn calls "informal meditation practice" to be more realistic than sitting in solitary meditation or going away on a retreat:

> We can bring mindfulness to any moment, no matter how brief or how stressed, no matter how off we may be feeling...mindfulness in everyday life is the primary practice we are recommending for parents. If you can also make formal meditation practice a part of your everyday life, even for relatively brief periods of time, say five or ten minutes a day, or longer, that of course can be extremely helpful in strengthening the muscle of mindfulness. But ultimately, mindful parenting involves dropping into the present moment over and over again and learning from this intentional opening into awareness.[135]

You can also practice in a "formal" way, which may be sitting meditation, writing, or some other mindfulness practice. Benefits of mindfulness can include decreased anxiety, connection with "the part of you that knows," and a sense of belonging with "common humanity." Dr. Kristin Neff, author of *Self-Compassion: The Proven Power of Being Kind to Yourself*, coined the term "common humanity" as one of the components of mindful self-compassion. About mindful self-compassion, she writes:

> When you feel compassion...it means that you realize that suffering, failure, and imperfection is part of the shared human experience.
>
> Self-compassion involves acting the same way towards yourself when you are having a difficult time, fail, or notice something you don't like about yourself. Instead of ignoring your pain with a "stiff upper lip" mentality, you stop to tell yourself "this is really difficult right now, how can I comfort and care for myself in this moment?"
>
> Instead of mercilessly judging and criticizing yourself for various inadequacies or shortcomings, self-compassion means you are kind and

understanding when confronted with personal failings – after all, who ever said you were supposed to be perfect?[136]

Motherhood is so full of tending to the externals of other people's needs. Spiritual practice can be a way to tune back into yours.

One Mom's Experience of Losing Herself in Motherhood (and Re-Finding Herself in Recovery and Spiritual Practice)

For the topic of spiritual practice and motherhood, I interviewed Jennifer Kreatsoulas, PhD, C-IAY, a mother of two girls, a yoga therapist specializing in eating disorders and body image, and co-author of *Body Mindful Yoga: Create a Powerful and Affirming Relationship with Your Body.*[137] Jennifer shared with me her journey of recovery from an eating disorder through finding yoga, and then re-finding her recovery and purpose through yoga years later. She taught yoga for seven years, prior to getting married and having children. After the birth of her second child, she went into treatment for her eating disorder after relapsing. Here is her story:

As painful as it was to leave my family and enter treatment, so many gifts came from that relapse. One is the work that I do now. I had the realization when I was in treatment that *if I'm going to be well as a mother, I need to be connected to my passions.* I need to have things in my life that make me feel like *me.* I had no idea who I was anymore. It's not that I didn't love my children – I adore them, and I would move mountains with my love for them. It had nothing to do with them. It was the fact that life had changed so much, and I needed to learn how to navigate that new world and allow myself to be in it. I needed to get back to writing, get back to yoga, get back to teaching yoga. And I needed to change my career, because my job wasn't my passion; it didn't fill me with a sense of purpose.

So much has come out of that relapse, and I thank God for it every day. I have so much new energy and purpose and passion! After the relapse, I came back to yoga. I got a few teaching gigs and, in the process of working with a life coach, I realized that my calling was to become a yoga therapist. So, I studied and trained for three years to be a yoga therapist, and it was in those years that I learned about yoga as a lifestyle. That's when I learned that yoga is always within me and with me. It's as simple as pausing to take a deep breath and connect with the moment, sensations, my children, and the world. That's when I learned the philosophies and all the ways that we can live our lives as an expression and practice of yoga. So now I don't have to go somewhere to "do" yoga. I can breathe when I feel like I am going to explode. I can keep myself grounded when chaos swirls around me. I can practice yoga as a tool to help me keep moving forward on my healing path.

Jennifer also shared about her current spiritual practice:

Right now, I don't feel like I have to go do it in a yoga studio. I try to get up a couple of minutes before everyone else, when the house is really quiet. That time is vital for my own sanity. I start my practice with some deep breathing and journaling. I ask myself, "What do I hear inside right now?" Or "What do you hear today?" Maybe I'm feeling grateful for my family, or I notice I feel hungry this morning, or I feel nervous about this, or excited about that. Just to have that moment of self-connection before I expend my energy connecting with my children, or my clients, or my husband [is vital and energizing].

She shares how these few minutes in the beginning of the day impact her, then, throughout the day:

> In the busy-ness of the day, in the craziness of the day, at the moment the kids are screaming and fighting, I give myself permission to believe it's OK that "I'm not perfect." I try to remember to take a few deep breaths. I try to remember that "reality is neutral." The screaming might be driving me crazy, but it's my reaction to the screaming that's really making me crazy. I can try to take responsibility for my reaction to things around me and be aware of what that reaction is before I act. I can understand that if that reaction is one that's not helpful to myself or people around me, I need to make sure I feel my feet on the ground and take a few breaths.
>
> Sometimes, I will pause, literally take three breaths, and wisely choose my words the best that I can before uttering them. I try to model awareness and calmness to my children. I try to model appropriate behavior. For me, yoga helps me do that. It helps me consider, when I make a mistake, maybe I could do it differently next time, instead of beating myself up. I don't have to say, "You're terrible." I get to practice compassionate self-study.

Here are some ways to fit spiritual practice in with the daily relentlessness of motherhood. *You do not have to do all – or any – of these!* Find what works for you. This is not an exercise in finding more ways to beat up on yourself for not doing enough or adding to the to-do list. The whole point is to cultivate compassionately objective kindness with yourself. Only you know how to do that in ways that will work *for you.*

Four Ways to Fit in Spiritual Practice between (or Right Along with) the Laundry and the Toys All over the Rug

1. RADICAL ACCEPTANCE AND "SPECIAL TIME"

When I practiced radical acceptance around not feeling like I was, or am, a good "floor mom," it opened up room for less judgment and more joy. Not ecstatic, exuberant joy, but a quieter, contentment-filled joy that comes with not fighting-what-is and trying to make-it-something-else. I didn't necessarily *like* playing on the floor with train tracks, but when I accepted this, it became not only easier, but even a little bit fun! I surrendered into playing with trains. And when I really put my full attention on playing trains with my little one, rather than thinking about all the things I'd rather be doing than playing trains, it was fun. Suddenly I was traveling on a train bringing supplies to the LEGO® people across the "country" (floor). There were several obstacles along the way…and even a traffic "jam" (jar of strawberry fruit spread, placed in between several Matchbox cars crashed along the train tracks) to get through… Before long, my little one and I were actually having a blast playing trains!

One way to practice this if you, like me, are "not a good floor mom" is what Hand-in-Hand Parenting calls "Special Time."[138] Special Time is a designated time each day when your child gets to decide what you are doing and playing. It doesn't have to be long – 10 to 20 minutes – which makes it manageable for the parent. But it does require your full attention. You need to be present. No multitasking, no bringing your coffee cup with you, and no texting-while-playing. Take a deep breath and, as much as you can, fully enter your child's world with them. Your child will most likely eat up this special attention that you give them. It is truly what most of us humans, regardless of how old we are, want: to be seen and to be loved for who we are.

You may even find relief from feeling like you never get anything done. (Have you ever noticed how anxiety-mind will always say, *"I'll go away once you finish everything on the list."* But then it keeps adding new items to the list?) Being present and slowing down often has a paradoxical effect on the part of you that would rather speed up and do more. Often, in eating disorder recovery treatment, I encourage clients to slow down, rest more, do less. If you are used to listening to the perfectionistic voice telling you, *"Do more"* and *"It is never good or never enough,"* this can feel excruciating at first. But please stay with it. Breathe deeply and practice witnessing this voice of "not enough" long enough to dis-identify from believing it to be the truth. Being present with yourself and your child are, perhaps, the only true way to have the experience of enough-ness.

The only rule with Special Time is: no hurting people or property. Other than no hitting, kicking, or punching (unless it's a pillow fight) and no breaking toys or furniture, the sky is the limit. You may find that your connection with your child deepens as a result of Special Time. You may find, like I did, that after Special Time your little one suddenly listens to you when you say, "No banging forks on the table" or "Please carry your dinner dish to the sink" or "It is bedtime now." Resistance tends to dissipate *if they are feeling the connection with and love from you.* And you both get to surrender the battle for control and just enjoy playing and connecting.

2. MINDFUL BREATHING AND RELAXING

Some simple (but not always easy) practices I do myself, and share with clients, include breathing mindfully, and systematically relaxing your body. One way to bring awareness to your breath is to count to four on the inhalation and count to eight on the exhalation. You can also notice how the air coming in the nostrils is slightly cooler on the inhalation and slightly warmer on the exhalation. The body warms the breath. Bringing awareness to the breath often causes a natural shift from chest-breathing, which is associated with being in your sympathetic nervous system (fight or flight), to abdominal breathing, which is associated with your parasympathetic nervous system (rest and digest).

Systematic relaxation involves bringing your awareness and attention to each part of your body, tensing and then relaxing it. You can bring your awareness to the top of your head, your forehead, all the tiny muscles in your face, scrunching them up and then relaxing and releasing them. Then do the same with your shoulders, arms, hands, and fingers. Continue tensing and then relaxing your abdomen, back, pelvis, thighs, lower legs, ankles, feet, and toes. Feel your feet on the ground. Feel the chair, bed, or floor supporting your body. For this one breath, breathe oxygen into all your internal organs, imagining them being massaged and relaxed by the breath, and on the exhalation, releasing any toxins that need to be released.

3. LOVINGKINDNESS

Lovingkindness meditation is a practice that uses words and feelings to evoke kindness toward oneself and others. It begins with bringing this kindness to yourself. As Jack Kornfield writes, and as every mother knows, "You begin with yourself, because without loving yourself it is almost impossible to love others." Breathing deeply and relaxing, this meditation includes saying the following phrases:

May I be filled with lovingkindness.

May I be safe from inner and outer dangers.

May I be well in body and mind.

May I be at ease and happy.[139]

If you want, you can place your hand on your heart while you say this to yourself. With each recitation of the phrases, express the intention to plant seeds of kindness over and over in your heart.[140] You may wish to imagine yourself as a young child or as you are now while you practice this lovingkindness. You can then choose to extend this love to your child, your spouse or partner, other moms, people in your life, the whole world.[141] If you have the time and the energy, you can then expand this intention of sending lovingkindness to those who feel easy to extend kindness toward (those you love), those you feel neutral toward, and those with whom you have a hard time extending kindness toward.

4. MOMFULNESS HUGGING MEDITATION

Denise Roy suggests doing a hug meditation at the end of the day, with family members, as a way to reconnect. Hug for three deep breaths: In, out. In, out. In, out. You may even discover that if you do this hug with your spouse or partner that your baby/children/pets feel that something wonderful is going on and want to join into a group hug.

> When you're first learning to do this, you may laugh or feel awkward. That's OK... Hugging is such a simple act. Yet when we feel held and touched and seen in ways that are far too rare in our busy lives, we realize that our bodies – and our spirits – are starving for that kind of touch.[142]

In Conclusion: There Is No Wrong Way to Practice

I'm going to repeat that you don't have to do any or all of these practices. They are simply ideas for ways to practice kindness with yourself in your motherhood and recovery process. You are allowed to practice them and discover what works for you and what doesn't. You are also allowed to practice different ones at different times. *You are not allowed to use these ideas as a way to beat up on yourself for not doing spiritual practice.*

Over the years in my recovery and motherhood journey, my concept of "God as I understand God" has changed, as have my spiritual practices. We are not static beings. If nothing else, motherhood teaches us *that!* Look at how your body has changed, and is changing. One of my first recovery mentors reminded me of the following (seemingly paradoxical) truths:

1. Change is the only constant

and

2. Repetition is the only form of permanence.

How can you embrace change? In what ways do you need the repetition of a practice in order to help be kinder, more compassionate, and more spacious with yourself and others? My wish for you is to find, again and again, practices that connect you with the part of you that knows. This is the best gift you can give your child: your self! In the words of Jon and Myla Kabat-Zinn:

> The greatest gift you can give your child is yourself. This means that part of your work as a parent is to keep growing in self-knowledge and in awareness. Can we be grounded in the present moment and share what is deepest and best in ourselves? This is a lifetime's practice. It can be supported by making a time for resting in awareness and in stillness and silence each day in whatever ways feel comfortable to us. We only have right now. Let us use it to its best advantage, for our children's sake, and for our own.[143]

9
Stay at Home Versus Working Outside the Home

—— ♡ ——

Discover the Right Balance for You, Right Now

Balancing motherhood with work takes experimenting, self-compassion, and re-evaluation. Be gentle with yourself. Remember: your value exists no matter what. It exists if you get paid for your work or you do not. It exists if you have a good day or a bad day. It exists if you feel connected to your children or not. Your value exists simply because you are a breathing, living human being, and each moment is an opportunity to begin again, and again, and again.

– Michelle M. Olsen, career purpose coach for moms and mother of two

What is the right balance between staying at home and working outside the home? Does staying at home with your kid(s) lead to greater emotional maturity for them as adults? Or does the opposite? What if you don't have the choice? What if you stay at home and hate it? What if you go back to work (outside the home) and it has lost its meaning? These are questions that all mothers wrestle with, to some degree. There is no "right" answer. Different sides in the "mommy wars" may think they have the right answer, and that can make it hard to live with the choices you make. As Leslie Morgan Steiner writes in her book, *Mommy Wars*, "Motherhood in America is fraught with defensiveness…and judgment about what's best for kids, family, and women – a true catfight among women who'd be far better off if we accepted and supported all good, if disparate, mothering choices."[144]

In my own experience, staying at home was much harder than leaving the house to work. When you leave the house to work, there are freedoms that come naturally that stay-at-home moms just don't have access to in the same way. A few of these perks are:

- Freedom to go to the bathroom *whenever you want, by yourself*, and without having to announce it or manage meltdowns as a result.
- Ability to eat your lunch without having bits of it snatched away or receiving already chewed bits of food that your child had decided they "don't like" spewed onto your plate.
- Having your colleagues respectfully listen to what you have to say, without yelling, "No!" or requesting, "Can we play cars/dolls/farm animals now?" in the middle of your sentence.
- Getting paid! With money!
- Not having to change any diapers, do any laundry, cook any food, mop any floors, sing any songs, or stay empathically listening during individuation-attempting tantrums for several hours.
- There is often time, on the way to or from work to stop for coffee, milk, or grocery shopping without having to redirect the child away from eye-level glittery treats. A ten-minute trip can actually take ten minutes!
- Quiet time. Yep. Work outside the home, post-parenthood, actually gets re-designated as "quiet time" or, as one colleague refers to it, "introversion recovery time."
- Intellectual stimulation and satisfaction.

As one mom puts it:

> I like to be engaged in the world, with a more intellectual, professional
> fashion than day-to-day childcare allows. I like the challenge and sense
> of accomplishment that work provides. I found that when I went for
> stretches without working, I really missed it. And, to be honest, I was
> bored silly by playing the same game for hours with the kids when they
> were young. As a friend put it, I'm not a great floor mom.[145]

The G Word

And the shadow side of working outside the home...? We all know
it: it's the G word. No, I'm not talking about God, here – much more
devastating for moms: *Guilt*. Guilt, along with anxiety, jealousy, and
angst, is one of the feelings mothers working outside the home wrestle
with most. A colleague of mine described her experience as a mom
who worked and had a nanny when her little one was a baby. Since
she worked from home, she would come out of her office at feeding
time to breastfeed. Her baby would reach for her and suckle until full,
then reach back toward the nanny to be held. She felt like the "wire
monkey" in Harlow's attachment experiments on infant monkeys.[146]
Dr. Melissa Arca, pediatrician and author of the blog *Confessions of a Dr.
Mom*, shared about her experience of working outside the home, and
poignantly quotes her six-year-old:

> "Mom, how come you don't take care of me that much?'"

> "Umm, what?"

> It's all I could choke out.

> And there it is, staring me right in the face. The guilt. In the form of big,
> beautiful, and earnest brown eyes. And I know exactly what she's asking.

Why am I at work all day? Why have I hired someone else to do my job? To care for her, feed her, soothe her tears, make sure she does her homework/chores, and mediate squabbles between her and Big Brother?[147]

When working with alleviating guilt for moms, I find it helpful to provide evidence for how it is not merited. Children of working (outside the home) mothers can and do thrive. Here is some evidence from a 2010 meta-analysis, published by the American Psychological Association:

> [Sixty-nine] studies over 50 years found that, in general, children whose mothers worked when they were young had no major learning, behavior or social problems, and tended to be high achievers in school and have less depression and anxiety.
>
> Employment was associated with higher achievement and fewer internalizing behaviors.
>
> The small effect size and primarily nonsignificant results for main effects of early maternal employment should allay concerns about mothers working when children are young.[148]

But What if My Child Is More Attached to the Nanny/Preschool Teacher/Grandma than Me?

Although all parents want caregivers with whom our children feel safe, it is a complex experience for a mom when her child reaches for the nanny/preschool teacher/Grandma, or acts uninterested upon Mom arriving home from work. For the record, this doesn't necessarily mean that the child is insecurely attached. Before you go into looking up attachment research on Dr. Google or pathologizing yourself as a "bad mom" who has created insecure attachment, *stop, now.*

I am going to remind you (or make explicit in a way that ... yet been made explicit) that the purpose of this book is to create a secure attachment for *you, the mother, inside yourself*, that you probably never had. If you have, or have had, an eating disorder, you are most likely trying to, or tried to, manage, comfort, soothe, or get rid of uncomfortable feelings of distress by using food (bingeing, purging, restricting, or obsessing). Why do you do this? You do this because you don't or didn't yet know another way to comfort, soothe, or manage uncomfortable feelings without using food (or obsessing about your body, exercise, anxiously reading parenting information on attachment styles). A secure inner attachment is the missing piece in knowing how to do this. It may not have been modeled for you. If your mother or primary caregiver didn't have it, s/he couldn't give it to you. And if you didn't get it, it is hard to give it.

All mothers want emotional security for their children. However, wanting secure attachment for your child does not mean you have to not work outside the home because you would be damaging your child for the rest of their life. Nor does it mean you have to be Mary Poppins all the time if you are staying home, in order to have a securely attached child.

Children can grow up in an "attachment village" where they can grow and thrive. If a child has a strong attachment, it can be to more than one caregiver. The times of Mommy-is-the-only-primary-caregiver are gone! In fact, "Married moms with children under 18 are now the primary breadwinners in 15 percent of households, up from 4 percent in 1960."[149]

No matter what work choice you make – whether by preference or necessity – you can have a secure child, and you can be a secure mom.

But how can you build this secure attachment inside yourself, so you can help foster it with your children? Along with the basics of self-care (showering, feeding, and sleeping), a secure internal attachment includes being fiercely and relentlessly kind to yourself when you are struggling. One of the practices I work with myself and with my clients is mindful self-compassion. Mindful self-compassion, a practice developed by Dr. Kristin Neff,[150] utilizes different practices to cultivate a kind caregiver voice inside yourself – toward yourself. One way to do this is to ask, *"Would I say this to a friend?"* If the answer is no, then ask, *"What would I say to a friend struggling with this?"*

Here is a personal example from when I went back to work. Though I desperately wanted to go back to work (being a new mom had leveled my confidence, and I welcomed returning to the work that I felt competent and qualified for), I also felt deeply ambivalent about leaving my six-month-old baby. The critical voice inside me said:

> *You are a bad mom for wanting to, and going back to, work. Your baby is going to be confused without you. And who is that person you hired? Do you even know her? I don't care how well you screened her; you should not leave your baby with her. You are supposed to be with your baby. You are being selfish going back to work. You say you're going to pump breast milk, but when and how are you going to do that? People are going to think you're slacking at work and asking for special treatment. Oh, and by the way, you probably will suck at work now, too. You will be too tired to have a clear head. And you have a mom-body now: **so** not-professional.*

As you can see, the content and tone of this self-talk is not exactly one of a kind caregiver. When I took a deep breath and was able to access the feelings I was experiencing in going back to work (sadness, ambivalence, excitement, fear) I was able to respond with a more loving voice.

> *Hi Honey. It's pretty scary for you to be leaving your baby after spending so much time with him. It's going to be OK. Of course you're scared! You are entering new terrain. You don't have any experience working outside*

the home and being a mom! I'll be here with you, through all the feelings and challenges as they arise. Just keep communicating with me, Honey. I'll stay with you when you're scared. I can help you strategize around finding a place to pump at work if you need that. Or if you need to let go of breastfeeding or pumping, that would be OK! You can still be securely attached with your baby. And as for the nanny: we'll see. I don't know how you could've screened her any more than you did. But if the nanny isn't a good fit, I will help you find another.

I don't think your worry is really about that, though. You are feeling scared about leaving your baby. I am here with you. Also, you can change your mind about going back to work right now. Even when it feels like you don't have choices, you have choices. I will stay with you through the fear. You can do this.

I had internalized the myth that *there is only one right decision, and once you make it you can't change your mind.* There are so many myths about motherhood that need fierce, compassionate challenging. Along with *you can never change your mind* come several more, about the choice to work outside the home.

Moms Should Only Work Outside the Home if They Have to (and Other Myths)

One colleague, a nutrition therapist mom, shared the following from her experience:

Over the course of my life, I had internalized a myth that moms only worked if they had to, which brought so much suffering and guilt when I realized I wanted to work.

Added to this myth, the work–life balance she had imagined did not end up being balanced at all:

When I returned to work, my husband and I made a mistake that colored the rest of my postpartum experience. To save money, we decided to only obtain childcare for the hours I was face to face with clients – one day per week – even though my true workload was closer to 30 hours per week. I was miserable. I couldn't appreciate the time with my son, because I was always trying to manage my business on the side. On paper, I had a dream life, but I felt anything but dreamy. I actually later learned I was dealing with postpartum depression and anxiety, and my work–life situation was a primary trigger. I remember thinking, "I started my business so that this part of my life would be ideal. How did I get here?"

As she assessed this imbalance, she obtained more days of childcare help, as well as adding the support of a therapist and psychiatrist for her own wellbeing. Moms need attachment villages, as well as children. Here are some of her learnings from using her own voice of self-compassion:

I learned to own the fact that I loved working, and to reject the idea that that fact said anything about how much I loved my son.

I learned to say to myself, "It's OK to want to work or want to stay home and to own that need and desire... Mute out all of the background noise and get non-biased support to help tap into what you really feel is best for you and your family. Your needs deserve to be met, because you are an inherently valuable human being, not just because you are caring for others. Seek out the support of a therapist in your postpartum journey!"

Closely related to the myth about working only if you have to is the myth that haunts so many mothers: *You Can Have It All!* The *You Can Have It All (and Never Feel Tired)* myth is one that causes suffering for so many moms. One colleague, a coach who supports moms in their transition back to work after becoming moms, shares about her own rocky experience:

> In my second pregnancy, I was super-fatigued and nauseous throughout, so the challenge was having the ability to show up for my clients. In hindsight, only by grace was I able to manage all my calls. Postpartum, with two kids, I was often overwhelmed, so integrating back into work was challenging at first. I had to figure out childcare, and then, of course, self-care. It was not easy. I am still working on it, to some extent, five years later.
>
> The "you can have it all" myth definitely had its grip on me. I was watching colleagues make big leaps in their coaching businesses, and I found I was judging myself often. Why couldn't I do that? What was wrong with me? What was I missing? Thankfully, I had a great therapist who helped me come back to myself and remind me, I was doing my best, and we all have different paths.

Her voice of self-compassion said:

> Be **gentle** and **trust your intuition**, not your inner critic but your inner wisdom. Rest, rest, and rest. Rest is sacred.

Another mom, a therapist who had to go back to work for financial reasons, shares the following:

> The worst part of going back to work was missing my kids. I would have loved to work four hours a day, not nine or ten. And working really was awful when the first nanny took over watching our kid. I struggled with many myths: "If you're not holding, touching, staring, and cooing at your kid, you are a bad attachment parent"; "You should love this all the time"; and "You should never feel anger at an infant."

I love her wise voice of compassion with herself that she shares, looking back on this time of early motherhood:

> *I am so proud of you. That was like being asked to be CEO of a Fortune 100 company with **zero** training. And by the way, your only job is to have as much fun being you-as-a-terrified-tired-grumpy-brand-new-mommy as you can. You can totally hate it some days. I celebrate you hating it. Throw a "f*ck it up party" because, my dear, that is so normal. And I think, the more you surrender to how lame these expectations are, the more you will have fun. Oh, and your kids are going to be fine. They are so wildly and incredibly resilient.*

Staying at Home Is Not a Pinterest Party

Just like working outside the home has its perks and challenges, so does staying at home. The obvious value is that a stay-at-home mom gets to be the one who is intimately involved with and witnessing all of the "firsts." One therapist mom shared:

> The best part of staying home was, I knew that I was not missing anything. I knew I would witness almost all developmental milestones. First word, first step, first wave, etc. Before both the kids were in preschool, I knew all that happened in the day, so I better understood where their emotions/behaviors were coming from.
>
> Staying at home allowed me to be very involved in my children's preschool. They would not have been able to attend a school that required so much parent participation if I had been working. Being a part of a community like this was so important.

However,

> I felt so trapped in my home: by pajamas, dirty dishes, and laundry.
> I needed to have a reason to go out to lunch and wear grownup
> clothes and to be my own person. I felt very depressed, isolated,
> and alone. I had spent so much time working on my career that
> I felt lost without it. I wasn't doing the work that I wanted to be
> doing. I had nowhere to go besides the coffee shop down the street.
> I felt smothered. My friends continued on in their lives, and I felt
> left behind. The days were brutal, long, and seemed to last forever...
> Then the baby came, and the oldest started preschool a few days a
> week, and friends started to have babies. This made me busy, and
> I felt less alone... The worst part has been not knowing what my
> future holds, losing confidence in my ability to be a therapist, and
> becoming very scattered in many ways.

Money, Power, and Value

Though free from the guilt of the working (outside the home) mom,
SAHMs have their own share of difficulties. One struggle I hear
frequently in the therapy office from SAHMs is feeling devalued
and disempowered in their work. Not getting a paycheck, not feeling
appreciated, and doing tasks such as laundry, changing diapers, mashing
peas, and picking goldfish crackers off the carpet around the clock
without being thanked can be trying, for even the humblest of us. One
mom shares her experience with her attempt to be "Donna Reed"[151]
after quitting her (outside the home) job and how she wrestled with
her new relationship with money and her husband:

Though my focus had shifted, I maintained an ambitiously busy life. I mothered lavishly, but on my own terms. I volunteered one morning a week in my daughter's first grade class... Life was as sweet as a 1950s sitcom. About six months in, the fantasy showed signs of strain, began collapsing under the weight of its lofty expectations – its disconnect with the salient facts of my life... I wanted to bring the girls to have their annual Christmas pictures taken, but my husband – saying we didn't have the money, and a nice Kodak would do just as well – vetoed it.

He vetoed it.

This was a notion that was unfathomable to me since I had always worked hard. I had a powerful memory of having money – which turned out not to be quite as powerful, actually, as having only a little bit of money. The strain of being wholly subsidized was beginning to take its toll. It was beginning to alter the power dynamic in my house. I had to plead and bargain and barter for things I used to be able to buy.[152]

Feminism and Killing the Myth of Supermom

Another separate, but related, issue of value and work (and devaluing women's work) is the cultural belief that "a woman's work is never done," which continues today. More than 20 years ago, Arlie Hochschild and Anne Machung began both conversation and controversy with the bestselling book *The Second Shift*,[153] which examines what really happens in dual-career households. Adding together time in paid work, childcare, and housework, they found that working mothers put in one month of work, per year, more than their spouses.

I have heard motherhood described as "the great leveler," meaning no matter what your experience prior to the actuality of motherhood, you will have many unforeseen learning opportunities, with no previous experience upon which to draw. Prior to motherhood, I worked as a nanny and at preschools, worked with moms in recovery from addiction and eating disorders, and held a doctorate in clinical psychology. And I was completely unprepared for motherhood.

The "shoulds" that often come with motherhood (I should know how to do this; I should have a plan for work postpartum; I should stick to the plan even if it's not working, because if it's not working that means there's something wrong with me; I shouldn't need help) are often painful. Women recovering from disordered eating tend to have an overdeveloped sense of perfectionism and a low tolerance for ambiguity and negative affect. In terms of work, this sets up many challenges, because these are the women who are therefore more likely to isolate, whether working inside or outside the home, and question whether they are doing it "right" or made the "right" choice. These are the women who may look good on the outside but feel as if they are falling apart on the inside. If they are staying at home, they only leave the house if they have their makeup perfectly applied before going to "Mommy and Me" classes. If they are working outside the home, they may be crying quietly in the bathroom, with feelings of guilt, insecurity, and grief, while breast pumping for the third time before returning to their boardroom to chair a meeting.

There Is No Right Answer: There Is the Right Answer for You, Right Now

Being a mom is a complex, difficult, rewarding, joyful, mundane, frustrating, ecstatic, and ever-changing job, regardless of whether one works outside the home or not. Childcare is a significant factor: whether you have extended family living near you who can help, what kind of childcare is available to you, what kind of childcare you can afford. In the United States, attitudes about working moms depend on the particulars of a family's circumstances, including whether they are happy with their childcare and whether they need the income. Here's what one *New York Times* article on working mothers says:

> The question is not just how working affects children, but how to deal with challenges like long and unpredictable hours and a lack of childcare.
> "Even in the U.S., where we continue to have this debate," Ms. Gerson [a sociologist at New York University] said, "we found that most people believe the right decision for a family is the one that works best for them."[154]

I repeat: being a mom is a complex, difficult, rewarding, joyful, mundane, frustrating, ecstatic, and ever-changing job, regardless of whether one works outside the home or not. I have no conclusions on what is "the right choice." The belief that there is a "right choice" is actually another myth of motherhood. SAHMs don't miss their babies' first steps, first words; they catch glimpses of discoveries that will never happen again. They often (*but not always*) have an easier time feeling confident that they are creating secure attachment and tending to their children's growth steps. *These things are priceless. There is no way to put a value on that.* And yet, it is not the right choice for every mom, and it is not a viable choice for every mom. One of my colleagues was a single parent protecting her children from their father, who had an untreated drug addiction. She separated from him and had to work outside the home to support the family. It wasn't a matter of what she wanted. It was a necessity.

I stayed at home for six months after having a baby. By the third month, I was starting to go stir crazy and afraid of losing my professional edge. But then, when I went back to work, I cried my way there. It got easier. (By the second week, I was loving it. My colleagues had gotten used to the sound of the breast pump and steering clear of particular milk bottles in the fridge.) It didn't get easier because I decided I'd made the perfect choice. It got easier because I came to peace with the choice I had made: and I re-made that choice, again and again. At six months postpartum, I went back to work two days a week. Then, later, three days… and then four. When my little one started elementary school, I shifted my hours to daytime, so I could be with him for dinner and bedtime.

There are strengths and weaknesses to any choice, just like there are pros and cons in any job. One colleague of mine went back to work full time when her baby was three months old. She is the executive director of her agency and couldn't take more time off. She regrets missing many of the first moments of her baby's development. She struggles with ambivalence, envy, and disdain for the moms who make their own Halloween costumes and homemade organic birthday treats. She also knows that she loves her work, needs the income to support her family, and wouldn't be happy staying at home. Another colleague is staying at home with her second child, who just turned two. She plans to go back to work (outside the home) when he is three. She doesn't love being home and admits to losing her sense of humor every single day, and she also wouldn't have it any other way. She wants to be there for her five-year-old as the room parent and for her two-year-old's formative years.

In Conclusion

Here is a good summary of how the process of deciding to stay home, not stay home, or stay home part-time can be an ongoing decision for moms over the years. Lydia Denworth, a journalist with three children, writes the following about her experience:

> As I prepared to have my first child, I chose to take a long maternity leave and then return to work. I assumed I'd do the same after the births of any other children I would be fortunate enough to have.

That's not how it worked out. In the eleven subsequent years, I have revisited that choice six times. I stayed home for a year. I worked part-time. I stayed home again. I worked full-time and then part-time and then full-time again. I have worked from home and from an office outside our house. I've also done a considerable amount of volunteer work.

I have had no help, a little help, and a lot of help with childcare. I have scheduled my life around pick-up and drop-off, and I have refused to schedule my life around pick-up and drop-off. I have used daycare, babysitters, au pairs, housekeepers, and after-school programs. I have my share of war stories from the clashing home and work fronts – like the day of a critical, impossible-to-reschedule interview, when one son had pneumonia and the babysitter had the stomach flu.[155]

Being a parent is a journey of ongoing decisions, again and again, none of them perfect, and all of them, hopefully, good enough.

If any woman thinks she is going to make only one decision – to work or not to work – she needs to think again. Because that is what she will actually be doing – thinking, again and again. It's never been just an either/or proposition. There are always additional questions like, "what type of work?" and "how much?" Paid or unpaid, it's still work.[156]

10
Advanced Maternal Age

———— ♡ ————

Navigating Life as an "Older Mom"

Sometimes I look around at the other preschool moms and I think, "I don't look like a new mom. I don't feel like a new mom." I LOVE being a mom. But I have middle-age wrinkles. I'm caring for my baby at the same time I'm caring for my ageing parents. I alternate between pushing a stroller and pushing a wheelchair.

– 44-year-old eating disorder survivor and first-time mother

When I went to my first ObGyn appointment, I saw my doctor write "AMA" on my chart. I said to her, "I am totally willing to be compliant with any medical recommendations you have!" She looked at me in bewilderment. I explained that in my profession "AMA" means "against medical advice." She smiled and explained that because I was over age 35, there were special medical considerations during the pregnancy, due to my being "advanced maternal age." "Oh," I stated, chagrined.

Being a mother of "advanced age" is becoming more and more common in developed nations, as women work toward completing higher education, solidifying their careers, finding the right partner, and doing personal growth work before having children. Some of the factors affecting a woman's choice to delay having a baby include effective contraception, gender equality, reaching higher educational levels, cultural value shifts, divorce or partnering later in life, lack of childcare support, an absence of supportive family policies in the workplace, economic hardship, job instability, or work in male-dominated fields that are not supportive of or understanding of motherhood.[157] Fertility treatments are another reason that people are getting pregnant later in life. According to Rebecca Dekker, PhD, RN, and her staff at Evidence Based Birth®, currently "15% of people giving birth are 35 and older, up from 11% in 2002 and 8% in 1990," and "10% of babies in the U.S. were born to first-time mothers age 35 or older."[158]

Women recovering from eating disorders often want to solidify their recovery prior to becoming a mother (for the record: recovery is often a process of years, not months), which can also delay the decision to conceive. Due to hormonal damage from the eating disorder and/or the decision to delay childbearing, many women with eating disorder histories attempt fertility treatment. By 2004, more than half a million babies had been born by IVF.[159] Becoming a mom at 35 (or older) comes with challenges that 22-year-old moms do not face. The cultural image of motherhood, looking young, glowing, thin, and unwrinkled, does not match the experience of middle-aged mothers. This sets up recovering moms to face a double whammy of transitions: motherhood and middle age. Although data regarding body image in middle-aged and older women remains sparse, a study published in *The International Journal of Eating Disorders* suggests that body dissatisfaction and drive for thinness do not diminish with age: 10 percent either suffered with subthreshold eating disorder or met the full criteria for an eating disorder.[160] Margo Maine, who co-wrote *The Body Myth: Adult Women and the Pressure to be Perfect*, writes:

> Women in their 30s, 40s and beyond face increasing pressure to look
> slender and youthful despite years of childbearing, hormonal changes at

menopause and the demands of careers, parenting and caring for ageing relatives... Some researchers call this the "Desperate Housewives effect" referring to the cultural influence of the hit TV series, in which improbably thin women in their 40s prance around in short shorts.[161]

There are many difficulties, especially for recovering women, with having a baby over the age of 35. And there are medical risks, too. I will say more about the risks now. But there are advantages, as well. I will talk more about them and share one woman's miraculous story later in this chapter.

What Are the Risks of Advanced Maternal Age?

Certain genetic risks are more common in pregnancies of older pregnant women. One risk is that the embryo will have Down syndrome, which happens when there is an extra copy of chromosome 21. The risk of having a baby with Down syndrome increases with the mother's age.[162] Risk of spontaneous miscarriage doubles from age 22 to age 35, and climbs to 84 percent by age 48.[163] High rates of miscarriage in older women are more related to egg quality than the physical ability to stay pregnant. Risk of stillbirth also rises with age of the mother.[164] Other risks, such as gestational diabetes, placenta previa, breech position, emergency Caesarean, and postpartum hemorrhage also increase with age.[165]

Is Being Older an Advantage?

Becoming pregnant over the age of 35 definitely carries risks. Advanced maternal age has consistently been associated with adverse pregnancy outcomes. But despite the increased risks, there are potential psychological and social advantages to delaying childbirth, and the absolute numbers of complications are small.[166] Jessica E. Tearne, in her review of the literature on older maternal age and child behavioral and cognitive outcomes, discovered "In contrast to the heightened physical risks for offspring, the existing research suggests that children of older mothers are often at lower risk for problem behavioral and academic outcomes compared with offspring of mothers in their teens and twenties."[167]

This makes sense to me as a mom and psychologist. As the executive function (part of the brain that has capacity to think in terms of cause and effect) does not fully develop until the late twenties, it would make sense that teenage and young mothers have not developed the capacity to regulate their own emotions and actions, much less those of a young child! Many of the twenty-something clients I work with are just beginning to be able to pause before using compulsive behaviors (overeating, bingeing and purging, drinking, shopping, etc.) to regulate their emotions. I, too, in my twenties was just beginning to figure out how to practice self-care.

Getting enough sleep, taking good care of yourself with food, hydrating, exercising moderately – all sound like simple activities of daily living. Pause when angry (if your tendency is to lash out), speak up when angry (if your tendency is to stuff your own voice and get depressed), also sound straightforward. Being kind (rather than critical and shaming) to yourself when you are feeling vulnerable, sad, or uncertain is a skill almost everyone I know would like to master (and hasn't yet). All of these skills are what 12-Step recovery programs call "simple, but not easy." In other words, most twenty-somethings are just beginning to identify these skills but are nowhere near mastering their implementation. And many thirty-, forty-, fifty-somethings are working toward mastering them, but still on the learning curve.

Having a baby will challenge even the most masterful of self-care gurus. In eating disorder recovery, we learn to prioritize self-care skills such as getting enough sleep, eating and exercising moderately, hydrating, communicating clearly with loved ones, meditating, etc. In motherhood, all of these areas are challenged. However, someone who has years rather than months or minutes of practice will likely have more resilience (and executive function) to ride the wave of these challenges.

Middle Age as Rite of Passage

Similar to adolescence, both parenting and reaching middle age are rites of passage in a woman's life. When not honored, seen, and embraced, such large life changes can also trigger eating disorders and body-image distress. Ageing women also face the cultural taboos of "taking up too much space," speaking too loudly, or not being seen and valued. They face the task of loving themselves and embracing aspects of the beauty of mortality, power, and wisdom that Western media culture is terrified of in women: wrinkles, thick middles, saggy boobs, gray hair. I remember reading one article on "objectification theory" in my doctoral research that linked media and female body-image obsession with Western culture's fear of mortality. Female body objectification may veil our unconscious existential fears.[168]

Another stress factor that affects women in middle age, similar to one that occurs in adolescence, is hormonal changes. Hormonal changes related to approaching menopause often include a slowing metabolism, weight gain, and shift in fat distribution around the middle. For women recovering from eating disorders, this can feel triggering. Difficulty regulating mood, body temperature fluctuation, and loss of libido can also be distressing. In addition, middle-aged women also face extra stressors such as medical scares, death of a parent or a spouse, divorce, and career challenges.[169]

A Hopeful Story

A dear colleague of mine had a baby at age 50. (Yes, that's right, 50.) I decided to include her whole story for this chapter on moms of advanced maternal age, as a source of experience and hope. Her name is Sheira Kahn. Sheira is a marriage and family therapist in private practice, with two decades of experience in treating eating disorders, three decades of her own recovery, and co-author of the book *Erasing ED Treatment Manual: Tools and Foundations for Eating Disorder Recovery.*[170]

Here is her eating disorder recovery, and becoming a mom at 50 story (personal communication):

> When I was a teenager and I was bulimic, the house where I lived was filled with turmoil that I literally couldn't stomach. Thankfully, when I moved out, I stopped purging.
>
> However, hatred of myself and my body persisted. I hated my body and I hated every bite of food that I ate. The mental part of the disorder persisted, though my physical responses had changed. I was in pain, and I knew that I didn't want to live that way. So I joined a meditation school where they taught us about how to work with the critic inside. And since my critic was always criticizing me about my body, I did what they suggested, to reduce the presence of the critic. Every time my inner critic was loud and mean, I practiced. And my relationship with my body changed, because there was less hatred being channeled from a critic toward myself. Then, a book on hunger and fullness signals taught me how to listen to my stomach, not my critic, when making food decisions. I later did 12-Step recovery in Al-Anon for relationship issues. In a way, you could say that my eating disorder – the root of it – had to do with these issues.

Did you always know that you wanted to be a mom or did that desire come later?

I always did, growing up, and then, in my twenties, I thought I didn't. And then, in my forties, it came back very, very strongly. I assumed motherhood would happen for me, as it seemed to happen so easily for other people. I had no idea that I would have to go through a lot to actually become a mom.

What happened?

For me it was a combination of factors. I wanted to be partnered. I married someone who I'd fallen in love with when I was 21. He wanted to have kids right away, and back then, I didn't. Then I changed my mind, but by that time, he had changed his mind!

That relationship wasn't working out for several reasons and we divorced. I was in my forties when I got married again, and started trying to get pregnant. I was on the late side, as far as fertility was concerned. It might have happened if I had felt safer in the relationship. However, I didn't feel safe in my second marriage to bring in a child. I believe this influenced my already shaky fertility. I would have had trouble getting pregnant anyway, but I think that feeling of lack of safety made me have even more trouble.

By this time, I really knew I wanted to have a baby, and I was ready to do whatever I needed to do. I wanted to have a baby, even without a partner. I just knew that I had to go for it. There were some things in place that showed me I could be successful being a mom. I felt healed enough in myself, I had a sense of inner strength, and I had support. And, I was making a good livelihood on my own at that point, so I knew I'd be able to provide for a baby. Knowing those things first had a lot to do with it.

What happened in the decade between 40 and 50?

I came from a family, in my childhood, where there was emotional trauma. There was extreme disconnection: fighting, antagonism, conflict, and fear – all the time. That gave me a layer of fear that I always carried with me and set me up to have very few skills for building long-term relationships. When there are emotional injuries like this, it's like a layer in your body – a layer of beliefs, feelings, and thoughts that went along with this fear. I thought that I would never be able to have a family. Or that it could happen for other people, but not me. I saw it happening for other people, and I believed that it couldn't exist for me. There was all this evidence I had that confirmed the belief I held: Sheira doesn't get to have family. I had been divorced once and was getting divorced a second time. I had miscarried.

It was important to make conscious those fearful beliefs and express them. When I touched in on those beliefs, I felt like throwing up. When I tried an embryo donation that fell through, I touched into this very deep grief about my family life not working out. It was a layer of grief that was so unconscious. It felt good for it to finally be out. That was one of the turning points for me.

I had another significant turning point specifically to do with my body. I had reason to believe I wouldn't be able to carry a child. I was afraid there had been too much damage done. I was telling this to a friend who's had three children. I was explaining how it wouldn't work out for me, and that I had evidence supporting this belief. She turned around and she said, "This sounds like depression."

She had a word for it. It was a relief to name it, this inner certainty, this layer of beliefs, as depression. It had only ever been the truth to me. And then she said, "Having children came really easily to me. Give your depression to me. I can help you with that."

And she did. She put her hands out and we kind of held onto

each other's forearms, and I just closed my eyes and said, "OK, I'll give it to you. I give you my depression about family." And she just accepted it; it ended there, in her unafraid psyche.

My fears finally had someplace safe to go. There was another human being who got in there with me. After that, I would still get fearful thoughts sometimes, but they just didn't have the hold that they once had.

And then some events happened that went counter to the evidence.

I got my mind around adopting an embryo, and I went on an embryo donation website. I decided on a certain set of embryos. There was a very expensive legal transfer of the embryos over to my possession. And, there was no legal precedent for transferring embryos. So, my lawyer had to basically do original scholarship on it. That required a lot of hours; it cost a lot.

And then, I met someone who was a much better-suited partner for me than the other two I had chosen. Finding my partner was a very important piece, although I had already made the decision to have a baby. I know other single mothers, and anyone who wants to be a single mother, I would encourage you to do that. I had to make the decision first, and then the right partner came.

How did your pregnancy go?

It took a while, but the embryos were transferred. Then I began the medical procedures that I needed to do. I was in full menopause in 2009 and I didn't get pregnant till 2014. I was 45 when I went through menopause. I think this was related to my eating disorder throwing off my hormones. Eating disorders mess up your hormones. Anyway, that's probably why I went into menopause early. My mother was 55 when she was in full menopause, and I was 45. If you have had an eating disorder, the good news is there's so much help now for both recovery and getting pregnant. It is all possible.

I got the green light from the head of the fertility department at UCSF that we could implant. It was an amazingly easy procedure. I had a very mild dose of the pain medication, and I was completely awake. There was a teeny, teeny, tiny tube that had the embryo in it, and they had to look at it with a magnifying glass to make sure the embryo was there! And then...then they put it into me, and then they checked with their magnifying glass that there was nothing in the tube and said, "That's great – it must be in there."

It felt like a conception. One of the members of the embryo donation family was there, and my partner was there, and a very dedicated acupuncturist. It seems futuristic and scientific, but that's how my baby got conceived. It was love. It was different, but it was still love. It was. It was not anything like I pictured, but it was still great.

My partner thought I must be pregnant, because she thought my boobs looked bigger. I didn't see any difference, and I did not feel any difference at the time. But I did a pregnancy test, and it came up positive. When I had been pregnant once before, I'd gotten really excited and happy and I felt like all my dreams would come true. I didn't feel that way this time. I felt simple, like, "Oh, this could happen."

Looking back, I realize that there was a knowing, but it wasn't like fireworks at all. I was afraid to get my hopes up. My whole world had been turned around as far as what I thought I knew about finding a partner, and what I thought I knew about how I would make my family.

It was very difficult with food. One way I recovered from my eating disorder was learning to eat when I was hungry and stop when I was full. But I didn't feel hungry when I was pregnant. I lost weight in the first trimester. I was getting worried, because I didn't think I was getting nutrition for my baby. I was at my "goal weight" of what I wanted to be – what I was in high school, in my eating disorder. I was so skinny! Why did I think that was attractive? I began to be concerned. I had to require myself to eat.

People were reassuring me that the nutrients for the baby would come from my body and I didn't have to worry so much about each bite. And, as the pregnancy progressed, the same people said the nausea was going to go away after 16 weeks. It didn't. It kept going, and I was worried. I was worried I was "carrying small." I went in and had a heart ultrasound. When the technician saw my ultrasound, she stopped the appointment to call the doctor and say, "We have a sixth percentile here." My baby was only in the sixth percentile of growth.

Now I became very worried. I was instructed to stop working in the office. I could still work, but I had to stay at home. I had been exercising. I was instructed to stop exercising. It was sad, because when I exercised I felt more able to eat, and I felt less nauseous. After that, I had to come in once or twice a week, just to make sure the baby was growing. By about a week before she came, I was in the normal range.

It's very unusual if you start out at the sixth percentile that you would get back into the normal range. I can't say exactly what happened. The doctor thought it was because I was working at home and stopped exercising. Clearly that helped. But it's still a mystery to me how she could have grown that much.

THE BIRTH

I told myself, "I'm never going to forget how painful it was." It's not fair to women that you don't remember it. This should be remembered. My beautiful baby came out, and she was strong. She was five pounds, eight ounces! At five pounds, seven, they take the baby into the NICU. She just made it. When they sewed me up, they were singing songs to her – for the last five minutes – it was very sweet.

My bonding with the baby didn't happen till the third day. I was really happy, and I loved her, but it wasn't complete bonding for three days. I thought I was going to have a completely empowered, expansive experience when I was giving birth. I thought my inner earth mother would come through me, and I would feel so competent! But my inner critic was there, huge and loud, every minute saying I was doing it wrong. That's the only voice I heard in my head. I was so surprised, and I was so pissed. After the birth, I heard them talking about me at the nurses' station:

"No pain medication?"

"Nope."

And then the nurse came in and she said, "You are my queen. I'm going to give you a tiara. All the other girls on this floor are 25 years old and they're asking for epidurals, and you came in here and you did your thing."

That was exactly what I needed to hear. I could not undo my own superego, and this lovely nurse did it for me.

This prompted a healing. I realized: I am in complete appreciation for all of my body. I can't believe I ever rejected it. And I realized that I had thought the hardware was flawed. I realized that the hardware was not flawed. It never was! The software was flawed. I believed that my body was incompetent, and I was wrong. My actual body knew what to do. My actual body is as beautiful as a tree or a flower in its infinite wisdom!

My daughter's name is Gracie. It's my way of thanking the family who donated the embryos and thanking God for finally giving me what I had wanted so much.

In Conclusion

This is just one woman's story. Please do not use it to "compare and despair." The intention is not to find the ways in which your experience is better or worse. (Reminder from Chapter 5 and the-part-of-you-that-knows: *everyone has their own pregnancy, labor, and delivery experience, and there is no "right" or "wrong" one*). Just take what is helpful from this story with you and leave the rest here in this book. I share her story here as a miracle of possibility: that you can create the life you want at any age. It may be difficult. Let me rephrase: it *will* involve difficulties. That is a given. Not to get too Buddhist on you, but life includes suffering. When you make choices that are aligned with your integrity, however, your recovery and motherhood journey may include more ease and joy.

I decided to have a baby at age 37. Before that I was a "No" for many years. Then a "Maybe" for many more. And then, at 37, I thought, *"This may not even be possible, but, Hell, Yes."* It was, and it is, possible. Becoming a mom is one of the most difficult, rewarding, and meaningful choices I have ever made. And the choice to embrace the choice of motherhood, with all its challenges, joys, and monotony, is a gift.

It is an interesting journey being "advanced maternal age." Sometimes I look at young(er) women or young(er) mothers and I think, *"You look so not tired."* Or, *"Wow, your stomach looks so not stretched. I remember that. That feels like a **long** time ago."* Or I envy younger moms who are more likely to have their grandparents be present for their children's growing up. My child will never meet one of his grandparents. He died before my baby was born.

However, there are gifts I have being middle-aged that I couldn't have come by earlier in my journey. I had not yet solidified my eating disorder recovery in my twenties. I had not earned a doctoral degree in psychology in my twenties. I had lots of really good ideas in my twenties that had not yet come to fruition and grounded-ness. (For example, I thought being earnest would pay the rent.) Interestingly, though I hated my (flatter) stomach in my twenties, I now love my (stretched) stomach in middle age. I also have much more capacity to pause and come back to difficult interactions in relationships rather than avoid, hide, or leave. I would not have had the "distress tolerance" skills to go toward a young child and stay emotionally present through individuation-attempting tantrums. I would have been inadvertently shaming or stuffed the discomfort with food. I can tolerate it now. I would not have been a good, or frankly even good enough, mother in my twenties. I wasn't ready. I remember studying for the psychologist licensure exam, learning that the executive function of the brain (the part that fully understands cause and effect and is able to therefore pause impulsive actions) is not fully developed until the late twenties, or even 30. Does that mean all women should only have children after age 35? Or that only women over 35 are good (enough) mothers? *Of course not.* One always has the potential to become a good (enough) mother. In fact, the eating disorder recovery process mirrors the journey of becoming a good enough mother to one's self: allowing and embracing imperfection, listening to and honoring emotions, communicating clearly, getting enough sleep, eating in a balanced way, practicing mindfulness or spirituality, connecting with support. *And **that** is always possible and always a work-in-progress, regardless of one's chronological age.*

The Good Enough Mama Recovery Pledge

I will not measure my worth on the scale.
Scales are for fish. I commit to not measuring my worth by the scale. I can throw out – or better yet bash and smash – my scale. I can bring my scale to my therapy session and have my therapist facilitate a break-up. I can tell my ObGyn and other providers that I want to be blind-weighed, and I do not want to have access to seeing my weight on my medical records. I can tell them I only want to discuss my weight if there is a *direct correlation* with a medical concern for myself or my baby. If I feel

anxious about my weight, or out of control, I can find other ways to tend to these feelings. I can put a deck of affirmation cards in the bathroom where my scale used to be.

I will listen to my body's hunger and satiety cues.

Whether I learned to listen for many years prior to becoming pregnant, or I am just starting the journey of listening, I can learn to listen to my hunger and satiety now. Instead of basing my eating choices on what, when, and how much I "should" eat, I listen to my body. I pay attention to what hunger feels like for my unique body, in this unique moment, with these unique needs. Just for this snack. Just for this meal. If I don't get it exactly right, I can try again at the next snack or meal time. I promise to keep listening to my body, not ignoring it, not restricting it, not stuffing it. I agree that fluctuating levels of hunger and satiety are part of having a woman's body, and these vary widely during pregnancy and postpartum. I commit to listening to these cues from a place of love, and a desire to take good care of my body and myself.

I will not try to do it alone. I will reach out for, and say yes to, support.

I will utilize my mom village for support. If I don't have one, I will create one. I commit to asking for – and receiving – support from my partner, other moms, my therapist, psychiatrist, doula, lactation consultant, family members. I realize that postpartum in particular is a time when I may be tempted to isolate. Isolating is different from needing introversion recovery time. I commit to listening to the-part-of-me-that-knows to discern this. I will set boundaries with people who are offering the kind of support I don't need (unsolicited advice or judgment). All new moms get overwhelmed and are in a massive learning curve. I commit to allowing myself to be in the messy soup of new motherhood, with support. I do not need to know everything ahead of time. I can be mentored and supported in learning to breastfeed (or not), swaddle, soothe, diaper, and tend to my baby. I am not supposed to do this alone.

I will sleep when I can, in the way I can.

My body and mind need sleep. This need is likely to be drastically impacted, and not sufficiently met, during pregnancy and postpartum. Instead of "shoulding" on myself around unsolicited advice ("You should sleep while the baby sleeps!"), I will find and create ways to sleep that work for me. If naps work, I will take naps. If I need to go to bed extra early and ask my partner to do the first nighttime feed, I will try that. If I need to stay up late and take the first shift for feeding, I will try that. If I need/am able to have my own mom stay or hire a night doula to replenish sleep debt, I will! I may choose to work with a sleep consultant for support. If I am sleep deprived, I can tell myself *this is a temporary window of time and it will pass.* If my mood is affected by sleep (too anxious to sleep or depressed from lack of sleep), I commit to prioritizing taking care of *my own* sleep as much as the baby's. I can ask for help and support with sleep: from my partner, therapist, family members, psychiatrist, doula, sleep consultant, friends. Sleep is essential. I commit to honoring sleep.

I will treat myself with as much kindness, respect, tenderness,
and fierce, protective care as I do my newborn.

I will practice talking to myself internally with a kind, non-critical voice. I will imagine a dear friend who is sleep deprived or struggling, and I will bring that quality of gentle compassion and fierce advocacy to myself. I will not shame myself. I am a brand-new mother, just like my baby is brand new. I have just as much to learn about how to be a mom as my baby has to learn about being a baby. I realize that I am not – nor is anyone – Supermom. Supermom is a myth. I do not have to be or feel glowing or competent. I will practice resilience and perseverance in the journey of new motherhood. If the voice of my eating disorder tries to come back and take over, I will separate from it, fight it, not believe it. If my critical voice says I am doing it wrong, or there is a "right" answer and I chose the wrong answer, I will remind myself there are no right answers. There is the right (good enough) answer for me and my family, right now. I will not give up on myself.

If I make a plan, I will be perfectly imperfect, implementing it.
Creating a birth plan, or a sleep plan, or a breastfeeding plan is important as a guide. I will realize *the baby has not read the plan.* If I make plans, I will do so with the intention of using them as a guide to help me, not proof of what a shitty job I am doing. I will look at the plan as something to work for me – not a dictator I am working for. I will use the plan as a structure when it is helpful and let it go or create a new one when it is not.

I will lower my expectations.
If I have bought into the myth of the perfectly made-up Pinterest mom who magically has all of her unfulfilled desires met through decorating the nursery and making her own organic baby food, I will challenge this myth. I will not expect myself to look like Instagram celebrity moms, who lose the baby weight (through dieting, hiring full-time trainers, and airbrushing photos) in three months. I will not compare and despair. I will lower the bar on expecting myself to accomplish what I used to accomplish every day, prior to having a baby. My main job as a newly postpartum mom is to rest. I will tell myself that I have many, many years to learn how to be the best mom I can be. I will tell myself it is OK to be in a learning curve, it is OK to feel uncomfortable, and there is nothing wrong with me.

The journey of motherhood can be difficult, easy, effortful, intuitive, and counterintuitive, just like recovery. Motherhood takes practice, support, endurance, surrender, and fierceness. I commit to staying on the journey. I commit to fierce compassion. I commit to being Good Enough.

Resources

——— ♡ ———

Below is a list of resources related to recovery that are meant to serve as support links for information and referral resources for treatment. The author does not endorse any specific treatment listed within these resources.

CRISIS LINES

United States

National Postpartum Depression Hotline: +1 (800) PPD-MOMS (773-6667)
Suicide Prevention & Crisis Hotline: +1 (800) 273-TALK (8255)

EATING DISORDER RECOVERY RESOURCES

United States

THE NATIONAL EATING DISORDERS ASSOCIATION (NEDA)
Nationaleatingdisorders.org
NEDA is a nonprofit organization that supports individuals affected by eating disorders and their loved ones. NEDA provides information, education, and treatment resources. The NEDA helpline is set up to provide support, resources, and treatment options for yourself or a loved one.
Helpline: +1 (800) 931 2237, Monday–Thursday 9 a.m.–9 p.m. (Eastern Time) and Friday 9 a.m.–5 p.m.

THE NATIONAL ASSOCIATION OF ANOREXIA NERVOSA
AND ASSOCIATED DISORDERS, INC. (ANAD)
anad.org
ANAD is a nonprofit organization that works for awareness, advocacy,
treatment, and prevention of eating disorders. ANAD offers support
groups, recovery mentors, and toolkits.
Helpline: +1 (630) 577 1330, Monday–Friday 9 a.m.–5 p.m.
(Central Time)

BINGE EATING DISORDER ASSOCIATION (BEDA)
bedaonline.com
BEDA is a nonprofit organization that works for recognition,
prevention, and treatment of BED and associated weight stigma.
Through outreach, education, advocacy, and weight stigma toolkits,
BEDA provides awareness and treatment resources for BED.

ASSOCIATION FOR SIZE DIVERSITY AND HEALTH
sizediversityandhealth.org
The Association for Size Diversity and Health (ASDAH) is a nonprofit
organization dedicated to the Health at Every Size® (HAES)
principles. The HAES movement works to promote acceptance of all
sizes and end weight stigma.

OVEREATERS ANONYMOUS (OA) AND EATING
DISORDERS ANONYMOUS (EDA)
oa.org and eatingdisordersanonymous.org
OA and EDA are 12-Step programs for people with problems related
to food including, but not limited to, compulsive overeating, bingeing,
purging, and restricting. They are low-fee, community resource
drop-in groups for recovery support. Because OA and EDA are
peer-led support groups, they do not offer professional treatment or

support that can be provided by a nutritionist, therapist, doctor, or psychiatrist. Any particular food plan followed in a 12-Step program is not endorsed by the author.

Note: 12-Step programs have a spiritual approach to recovery. If you are looking for a secular support group, please see the resources listed above or contact your local eating disorder treatment program(s), as many offer community groups or can refer you to a therapist-led, secular support group.

Canada

NATIONAL EATING DISORDER INFORMATION CENTRE (NEDIC)

nedic.ca

NEDIC is an organization that supplies outreach, information, and educational programs for the treatment and prevention of eating disorders.

Toll-free helpline: +1 (866) 633 4220

NATIONAL INITIATIVE FOR EATING DISORDERS (NIED)

nied.ca

NIED creates awareness and understanding through free educational symposia presented by experts in the field. NIED also works to address the gaps and delays in current treatment as well as training for professionals. NIED advocates for including eating disorders in mental health discussions, policies, organizations, programs, and campaigns.

United Kingdom

BEAT

Beateatingdisorders.org.uk

Beat, formerly the Eating Disorders Association, is a UK eating disorder charity that offers information, advocacy, support services,

and awareness trainings on recovery. In addition, Beat offers a HelpFinder service to assist people in finding treatment in their area. Beat offers additional resources such as message boards, online support groups, and regional support services.
Helpline: 0808 801 0677, 3 p.m.–10 p.m. daily

Australia

THE BUTTERFLY FOUNDATION
thebutterflyfoundation.org.au
Butterfly Foundation offers services that provide support, treatment, prevention, early intervention, education, and training on eating disorders. In addition, the Butterfly Foundation offers a national helpline.
Helpline: 1800 334673

PERINATAL MOOD DISORDER RESOURCES

POSTPARTUM SUPPORT INTERNATIONAL (PSI)
postpartum.net
PSI was created to increase awareness about perinatal mood disorders that women and men can experience during pregnancy and postpartum. PSI shares information and resources through its volunteer coordinators, website, and annual conference. It provides a wealth of information and online support, as well as advocates for research and legislation to support perinatal mental health.
Toll-free helpline: +1 (800) 944 4PPD (4773), refers callers to appropriate local resources, including emergency services

POSTPARTUM PROGRESS
postpartumprogress.com
Postpartum progress is a blog dedicated to maternal mental illness

and recovery. The blog offers information, support, and hope for pregnant and new moms who experience perinatal mood disorders, including anxiety, depression, bipolar, OCD, or psychosis. **Note:** This resource is a blog, not a treatment or referral service.

SELINI INSTITUTE

seleni.org

The Seleni Institute is a nonprofit organization supporting the emotional health of individuals and families during the early parenting years. Selini offers services and support on a broad range of topics including (but not limited to) infertility, miscarriage, and perinatal mood disorders.

United Kingdom

THE MARCÉ SOCIETY FOR PERINATAL MENTAL HEALTH

marcesociety.com

The Marcé Society is an organization that supports research and assistance surrounding perinatal mental health for mothers, fathers, and their babies. The Marcé Society aims to support and communicate research on all aspects of the mental health of women, their infants, and partners around the time of childbirth.

Canada

POSTPARTUM EDMONTON

PostPartumEdmonton.com

Postpartum Edmonton is a comprehensive website with resources for mothers and fathers experiencing mood disorders during pregnancy or postpartum. It also has resources for professionals and supporting families.

Australia

THE CENTRE OF PERINATAL EXCELLENCE (COPE) IN AUSTRALIA

cope.org.au

COPE is a nonprofit organization dedicated to providing evidence-based information, research, and advocacy to improve quality of life for those living with mental health challenges during the perinatal period.

SURVIVORS OF SEXUAL TRAUMA

WHEN SURVIVORS GIVE BIRTH

whensurvivorsgivebirth.net

When Survivors Give Birth is a book written by Penny Simkin, PT and Phyllis Klaus, MFT, LCSW (Seattle, WA: Classic Day Publishing, 2004) for women survivors of sexual abuse. This book helps with understanding and healing the effects of sexual abuse on childbearing women for survivors and their maternity caregivers. The When Survivors Give Birth website is a resource that lists facilitators who have been trained to help survivor women.

RESOURCES FOR HUSBANDS AND PARTNERS

POSTPARTUMMEN.COM

Men get postpartum depression, too. Postpartum Men provides information for fathers, including a self-assessment for postpartum depression. Postpartum Men offers an online forum for dads to talk to each other and provides resources.

THE POSTPARTUM HUSBAND: PRACTICAL SOLUTIONS
FOR LIVING WITH POSTPARTUM DEPRESSION

The Postpartum Husband (Bloomington, IN: XLibris, 2000) is a book written by Karen Kleiman, MSW. This hands-on guide includes straightforward information and specific recommendations to help husbands/partners support a wife/mom with postpartum depression.

CONFESSIONS OF THE OTHER MOTHER
Confessions of the Other Mother is a book by Harlyn Aizley (Boston, MA: Beacon Press, 2006). In it you will find a collection of stories shared by women who are in the process of creating new parenting roles and reshaping our view of two-parent families.

MOMMIES, DADDIES, DONORS, SURROGATES: ANSWERING
TOUGH QUESTIONS AND BUILDING STRONG FAMILIES
Mommies, Daddies, Donors, Surrogates (New York, NY: Guilford Press, 2005) is a book by Dr Diane Ehrensaft, a clinical psychologist who has worked with families using reproductive technology for over 20 years. Anyone looking for information or support on the many questions that arise when building a family with the help of a donor or surrogate is likely to find practical information in this book.

INFERTILITY

RESOLVE
resolve.org
RESOLVE, The National Infertility Association, provides access to care, advocacy for coverage, support, and education for anyone struggling with infertility.

ADVANCED MATERNAL AGE
advancedmaternalage.org
Advanced Maternal Age is a nonprofit organization that is working toward providing resources, information, and a safe place to share their stories for women having children at the age of 35 or over.

MEDICATION DURING PREGNANCY/ BREASTFEEDING

DR. THOMAS HALE, MEDICATIONS AND MOTHERS' MILK

medsmilk.com

Medications and Mothers' Milk Online (MMM Online) includes information from the book *Medications and Mothers' Milk* by Thomas W. Hale, PhD (New York, NY: Springer Publishing, 2017). The book and website provide information regarding medication use in breastfeeding mothers. The information provided is intended to supplement, not replace, treatment and clinical judgment and individual care from healthcare professionals.

MOTHERTOBABY

Mothertobaby.org

MotherToBaby provides evidence-based information about medications and other exposures during pregnancy and while breastfeeding. Information is available to mothers, healthcare professionals, and the public.

PREGNANCY AND INFANT LOSS

SHARE PREGNANCY AND INFANT LOSS SUPPORT

nationalshare.org

Share Pregnancy and Infant Loss Support is a community for people who have experienced the death of a baby. Their services include (but are not limited to) support by phone or bedside, in-person support, groups, resource packets, online communities, memorial events, and training for caregivers.

Endnotes

——— ♡ ———

Chapter 1

1   Norwegian Institute of Public Health, "Pregnant women with bulimia have more anxiety and depression, study finds," *ScienceDaily*, September 18, 2008, www.sciencedaily.com/releases/2008/09/080917095356.htm

2   B.N. Gaynes, N. Gavin, S. Meltzer-Brody, K.N. Lohr, T. Swinson, and G. Gartlehner, *Perinatal Depression: Prevalence, Screening Accuracy, and Screening Outcomes* (Rockville, MD: Agency for Healthcare Research and Quality, US Department of Health and Human Services), https://archive.ahrq.gov/downloads/pub/evidence/pdf/peridepr/peridep.pdf

3   K.L. Wisner, D.K. Sit, M.C. McShea, D.M. Rizzo, *et al.*, "Onset timing, thoughts of self-harm, and diagnosis in postpartum women with screen-positive depression findings," *JAMA Psychiatry 70*, 5 (2013): 490–498.

4   April Hirschberg, "Postpartum depression and poor sleep quality occur together," Massachusetts General Hospital Center for Women's Mental Health, June 6, 2011, https://womensmentalhealth.org/posts/postpartum-depression-and-poor-sleep-quality-occur-together

5   Intuitive eating incorporates principles such as rejecting the diet mentality, honoring your hunger, satisfaction, and fullness, and making peace with food. *Intuitive Eating: A Revolutionary Program that Works* by Evelyn Tribole and Elyse Resch (Manhattan, NY: St. Martin's Press, originally published in 1995, updated 2012) is the book from which these principles were taken.

6   Health at Every Size and HAES are registered trademarks of the Association for Size Diversity and Health (ASDAH) and are used with permission. ASDAH is an international professional organization composed of members committed to the Health at Every Size (HAES) principles.

The book *Health at Every Size: The Surprising Truth About Your Weight* (Dallas, TX: BenBella Books, 2010) by Linda Bacon empirically challenges many assumptions such as that anyone who is determined can lose weight and keep it off, and that health is declining with the "obesity epidemic."

It encourages challenging messages from the economics of diet culture and encourages accepting your body's natural size and trusting yourself as a radical form of not only self-love, but also social justice.

7   World Health Organization, "Breastfeeding," www.who.int/topics/breastfeeding/en

8   See www.dbtselfhelp.com/html/overview1.html. Dr. Marsha Linehan, the developer of dialectical behavior therapy, is a professor of psychology and an adjunct professor of psychiatry at the University of Washington. She is also the director of the Behavioral Research and Therapy Clinics, where she conducts research to develop and evaluate treatments for severe and complex mental disorders. www.dbtselfhelp.com/html/overview1.html

9   Eating Disorders Resource Catalogue, "Yoga and Eating Disorders: Ancient Healing for Modern Illness Interview," October 31, 2016, www.edcatalogue.com/yoga-eating-disorders-ancient-healing-modern-illness-interview

10 Two books that address maternal ambivalence are: Barbara Almond, *The Monster Within* (Berkeley, CA: University of California Press, 2011) and Jill Smokler, *Motherhood Comes Naturally: And Other Vicious Lies* (New York, NY: Gallery Books, 2013).

11 *The Second Shift* (New York: Penguin, 2003), by Arlie Hochschild and Anne Machunga, updated in 2003 and 2012, found that women working outside the home also work an extra *month* of 24-hour days over the course of the year doing child-rearing and housework-related tasks.

12 T.J. Mathews and Brady E. Hamilton, *Delayed Childbearing: More Women Are Having Their First Child Later in Life*, Centers for Disease Control and Prevention NCHS Data Brief, Number 21, August 2009, www.cdc.gov/nchs/data/databriefs/db21.htm

13 B. Mangweth-Matzek, H.W. Hoek, C.I. Rupp, K. Lackner-Seifert, *et al.*, "Prevalence of eating disorders in middle-aged women," *International Journal of Eating Disorders 47*, 3 (2014): 320–324.

14 Pema Chodron, *The Places that Scare You: A Guide to Fearlessness in Difficult Times* (Boston, MA: Shambhala Publications, 2001).

15 William Stafford, *The Way It Is: New and Selected Poems* (Minneapolis, MN: Graywolf Press, 1999).

16 D.L. Norris, "The effects of mirror confrontation on self estimation of body dimensions in anorexia nervosa, bulimia, and two control groups," *Psychological Medicine 14* (1984): 835–842.

17 Peter David Slade, "What is body image?" *Behavioral Research Therapy 32*, 5 (1994): 497–502.

18 Ibid.

19 Jean Hersholt, "The Emperor's New Clothes: A translation of Hans Christian Andersen's 'Keiserens Nye Klæder,'" The Hans Christian Andersen Centre, www.andersen.sdu.dk/vaerk/hersholt/TheEmperorsNewClothes_e.html

20 Marsha M. Linehan, PhD is the originator of dialectical behavioral therapy, and is a professor of psychology and an adjunct professor of psychiatry at the University of Washington. She is also the director of the Behavioral Research and Therapy Clinics, where she conducts research to develop and evaluate treatments for severe and complex mental disorders. Her most recent skills workbook is the *DBT Skills Training Manual* (second edition; New York, NY: Guilford Press, 2014). See https://behavioraltech.org/about-us/founded-by-marsha

21 J.P. Ogle, K. Tyner, and S. Schofield-Tomschin, "Jointly navigating the reclamation of the 'woman I used to be': Negotiating concerns about the postpartum body within the marital dyad," *Clothing and Textiles Research Journal 29*, 1 (2011): 35–51.

22 Anne Lamott, *Traveling Mercies: Some Thoughts on Faith* (New York: Random House, 1999).

Chapter 2

23 Karen Kleiman and Valerie D. Raskin, *This Isn't What I Expected* (Boston, MA: Da Capo Press, 2013).

24 Shawn Bean, "Xanax makes me a better mom," *Parenting Magazine*, March 2013.

25 K.L. Wisner, D.K. Sit, M.C. McShea, D.M. Rizzo, et al., "Onset timing, thoughts of self-harm, and diagnoses in postpartum women with screen-positive depression findings," *JAMA Psychiatry 70*, 5 (2013): 490–498.

26 S.E. Mazzeo, M.C. Slof-Op't Landt, I. Jones, K. Mitchell, et al., "Associations among postpartum depression, eating disorders, and perfectionism in a population-based sample of adult women," *International Journal of Eating Disorders 39*, 3 (2006): 202–211.

27 S.A. Swanson, S.J. Crow, D. Le Grange, J. Swendsen, and K.R. Merikangas, "Prevalence and correlates of eating disorders in adolescents: Results from the National Comorbidity Survey Replication Adolescent Supplement," *Archives of General Psychiatry 68*, 7 (2011): 714–723.

28 J.E. Steinglass, R. Sysko, L. Mayer, L.A. Berner, et al., "Pre-meal anxiety and food intake in anorexia nervosa," *Appetite 55*, 2 (2010): 214–218.

29 A.A. Haedt-Matt and P.K. Keel, "Revisiting the affect regulation model of binge eating: A meta-analysis of studies using ecological momentary assessment," *Psychological Bulletin 137*, 4 (2011): 660–681.

30 Shoshana Bennett and Pec Indman, *Beyond the Blues: A Guide to Understanding and Treating Prenatal and Postpartum Depression* (San Jose, CA: Moodswings Press, 2003).

31 Ibid.

32 Katherine Stone, "The symptoms of postpartum depression & anxiety (in plain mama English)," Postpartum Progress, www.postpartumprogress.com/the-symptoms-of-postpartum-depression-anxiety-in-plain-mama-english

33 Postpartum Support International, "Postpartum Psychosis Help," www.postpartum.net/get-help/postpartum-psychosis-help

34 Sutter Health CPMC, "Postpartum Depression," The Women's Health Resource Center, www.cpmc.org/services/women/health/postpartum-blues.html

35 Brooke Shields, "War of Words," *New York Times Opinion*, July 1, 2005, https://www.nytimes.com/2005/07/01/opinion/war-of-words.html

36 Ibid.

37 Brooke Shields, "War of Words," *New York Times Opinion*, July 1, 2005, https://www.nytimes.com/2005/07/01/opinion/war-of-words.html

38 Maria Yagoda, "Serena Williams, Alyssa Milano, Lena Headey, Chrissy Teigen & more stars who've opened up about their struggles with postpartum depression," People, May 31, 2018.

39 The Blue Dot Project, "This May, Angelina Spicer and TheBlueDotProject are asking moms to #GetReal," *Cision PR Newswire*, April 19, 2018, www.prnewswire.com/news-releases/this-may-angelina-spicer-and-thebluedotproject-are-asking-moms-to-getreal-300632820.html

  The Blue Dot Project is a project of 2020 Mom. The Blue Dot symbol, a blue circle, was inspired by a robin's egg and represents solidarity and maternal mental health awareness. 2020 Mom is an organization committed to closing gaps in maternal mental health care. www.thebluedotproject.org

40 Thomas W. Hale, "About," Medication and Mother's Milk Online, www.medsmilk.com/pages/about

41 Postpartum Support International is a fabulous resource to start if you are looking for support resources: Postpartum.net

42 Norwegian Institute of Public Health, "Pregnant women with bulimia have more anxiety and depression, study finds," *Science Daily*, September 18, 2008, www.sciencedaily.com/releases/2008/09/080917095356.htm

43 Decker Cline, "Does weight gain during pregnancy influence postpartum depression?" *Journal of Health Psychology* 17 (2012): 333–342.

44 Ngozi Onunaku, *Improving Maternal and Infant Mental Health: Focus on Maternal Depression* (Los Angeles, CA: National Center for Infant and Early Childhood Health Policy at UCLA, 2005). Available at www.zerotothree.org/resources/137-improving-maternal-and-infant-mental-health-focus-on-maternal-depression

45 C.W. Fu, J.T. Liu, W.J. Tu, J.Q. Yang, and Y. Cao, "Association between serum 25-hydroxyvitamin D levels measured 24 hours after delivery and postpartum depression," *BJOG: International Journal of Obstetrics and Gynaecology 122*, 12 (2015): 1688–1694.

46 Crappypictures.com

47 Jill Smokler, *Motherhood Comes Naturally: And Other Vicious Lies* (New York, NY: Gallery Books, 2013).

48 Scarymommy.com/category/PPD

49 Katherine Stone, "The symptoms of postpartum depression & anxiety (in plain mama English)," Postpartum Progress, www.postpartumprogress.com/the-symptoms-of-postpartum-depression-anxiety-in-plain-mama-english

50 Thomas Moore, *Care of the Soul* (New York, NY: HarperCollins, 1992).

Chapter 3

51 Kelly Bulkeley, "Why sleep deprivation is torture," *Psychology Today*, December 15, 2014.

52 Thomas Roth and Sonia Ancoli-Israel, "Daytime consequences and correlates of insomnia in the United States: Results of the 1991 National Sleep Foundation Survey, II." *Sleep: Journal of Sleep Research & Sleep Medicine* 22 (1999): S354–S358.

53 P.H. Finan, P.J. Quartana, and M.T. Smith, "The effects of sleep continuity disruption on positive mood and sleep architecture in healthy adults," *Sleep 38*, 11 (2015): 1735–1742.

54 For a beautiful version of Brené Brown's Parenting Manifesto, see https://brenebrown.com/wp-content/uploads/2013/09/DaringGreatly-ParentingManifesto-light-8x10.pdf

55 Dr. Sears (and his wife, Martha, and son, James) are best known for their book *The Baby Book* (third edition; Boston, MA: Little, Brown and Company, 2013), which covers many different parenting topics from the perspective of attachment parenting.

56 Dr. Richard Ferber is a physician and the director of The Center for Pediatric Sleep Disorders at Children's Hospital Boston, best known for his book *Solve Your Child's Sleep Problems* (New York, NY: Fireside Books, 2006).

57 Kate Pickert, "The man who remade motherhood." *Time Magazine*, May 21, 2012.

58 Ibid.

59 Allan Coukell, "Dr. Ferber revisits his 'crying baby' theory," National Public Radio interview, May 30, 2006.

60 Ibid.

61 Gwen Dewar, "The Ferber method: What does the evidence tell us about 'cry it out' sleep training?" Parenting Science, 2017, www.parentingscience.com/Ferber-method.html

62 Ibid.

63 Ibid.

64 Allan Coukell, "Dr. Ferber revisits his 'crying baby' theory," National Public Radio interview, May 30, 2006.

65 sleepfoundation.org

66 M. Robinson, A.J. Whitehouse, J.P. Newnham, S. Gorman, *et al.*, "Low maternal serum vitamin D during pregnancy and the risk for postpartum depression symptoms," *Archives of Women's Mental Health 17*, 3 (2014): 213–219.

Chapter 4

67   For more information on HAES principles, please visit the Association for Size Diversity and Health (ASDAH) website, www.sizediversityandhealth.org/content.asp?id=76

68   Linda Bacon, *Health at Every Size: The Surprising Truth about Your Weight* (Dallas, TX: BenBella Books, 2010).

69   Laura Hill, PhD, citing her own work and the work of Walter H. Kaye and Christina E. Wierenga at the 2018 International Association of Eating Disorder Professionals (IAEDP) Conference, Neuroscience: Magic of the Mind and Language of the Body, "Nourishing neurons: Brain-based nutrition therapy for eating disorders," Orlando, Florida, March 22–25, 2018.

70   Rosanna Franklin, PsyD, *You Are (Not) What Your Mother Eats: Maternal Intuitive Eating and Perceptions of Child's Eating*, Thesis, Alliant International University, 2015.

71   Myles S. Faith, Kelley S. Scanlon, Leann L. Birch, Lori A. Francisci, and Bettylou Sherry, "Parent–child feeding strategies and their relationships to child eating and weight status," *Obesity Research 12*, 11 (2004): 1711–1722.

72   Leslie A. Frankel, Sheryl O. Hughes, Teresia M. O'Connor, Thomas G. Power, Jennifer O. Fisher, and Nancy L. Hazen, "Parental influences on children's self-regulation of energy intake: Insights from developmental literature on emotion regulation," *Journal of Obesity* (2012), doi: 10.1155/2012/327259.

73   Ellyn Satter, "Raise a healthy child who is a joy to feed," Ellyn Satter Institute, www.ellynsatterinstitute.org/how-to-feed/the-division-of-responsibility-in-feeding.

      Ellyn Satter, MS, RD, LCSW, BCD is an internationally recognized authority on eating and feeding. A family therapist and feeding and eating specialist, she developed the "division of responsibility in feeding." Dr. Satter is the author of several eating-related books, including *Child of Mine: Feeding with Love and Good Sense* (Boulder, CO: Bull Publishing, 2000) and *Secrets of Feeding a Healthy Family: How to Eat, How to Raise Good Eaters, How to Cook* (Madison, WI: Kelcy Press, 2008).

74   More on Ellyn Satter (and downloadable handouts) here: http://ellynsatterinstitute.org

75   F. Grodstein, R. Levine, T. Spencer, G.A. Colditz, and M.J. Stampfer, "Three-year follow-up of participants in a commercial weight loss program: Can you keep it off?" *Archives of Internal Medicine 156*, 12 (1996): 1302–1306.

76   D. Neumark-Sztainer, *I'm, Like, SO Fat!* (New York, NY: Guilford, 2005).

77   C.M. Shisslak, M. Crago, and L.S. Estes, "The spectrum of eating disturbances," *International Journal of Eating Disorders 18*, 3 (1995): 209–219.

78   Evelyn Tribole and Elyses Resch, *Intuitive Eating: A Revolutionary Program that Works* (third edition; New York, NY: St. Martin's Griffin, 2012).

79 *The Onion*, "Mom's bathing suit just one giant, body-eclipsing ruffle," August 25, 2014, www.theonion.com/mom-s-bathing-suit-just-one-giant-body-eclipsing-ruffl-1819591849

80 Ellyn Satter, "Raise a healthy child who is a joy to feed," Ellyn Satter Institute, www.ellynsatterinstitute.org/how-to-feed/the-division-of-responsibility-in-feeding

81 Brené Brown, *Daring Greatly: How the Courage to Be Vulnerable Transforms the Way We Live, Love, Parent, and Lead* (New York, NY: Avery, 2015).

82 Oprah Winfrey Network interview, "Brené Brown on shame: 'It cannot survive empathy,'" *Huffington Post*, August 26, 2013, www.huffingtonpost.com/2013/08/26/brene-brown-shame_n_3807115.html

Chapter 5

83 Pam England and Rob Horowitz, *Birthing from Within: An Extra-Ordinary Guide to Childbirth Preparation* (Albuquerque, NM: Partera Press, 1998).

84 Ibid.

85 Britt Fohrman is a birth doula, prenatal yoga teacher, and pregnancy/birth photographer in the San Francisco Bay area. Learn more at www.Brittfohrman.com

86 With an online nutrition practice, Crystal Karges, MS, RDN, IBCLC, helps mamas and their families nurture a peaceful relationship with food and their bodies to experience the abundance of motherhood and truly thrive in life. Learn more at www.crystalkarges.com

87 Leora Fulvio is a master's level psychotherapist in the San Francisco Bay area. She offers psychotherapy to adults and adolescents, couples and families, and specializes in treating eating disorders. To learn more about her, visit www.leorafulvio.com

88 Augmentation = intervention to stimulate contractions; amniotomy = artificial rupture of the membrane (sometimes referred to as AROM) of the amniotic sac to induce or accelerate labor; Pitocin® = a synthetic form of oxytocin used to induce labor.

89 J. Sandall, H. Soltani, S. Gates, A. Shennana, and D. Devane, "Midwife-led continuity models versus other models of care for childbearing women," *Cochrane Database of Systematic Reviews* 4 (2016), doi: 10.1002/14651858.CD004667.pub5

90 A.R. Kroll-Desrosiers, B.C. Nephew, J.A. Babb, Y. Guilarte-Walker, T.A. Moore Simas, and K.M. Deligiannidis, "Association of peripartum synthetic oxytocin administration and depressive and anxiety disorders within the first postpartum year," *Depression and Anxiety* 34, 2 (2017): 137–146.

91 Kathleen Kendall-Tackett, Zhen Cong, and Thomas W. Hale, "Birth interventions related to lower rates of exclusive breastfeeding and increased risk of postpartum depression in a large sample," *Clinical Lactation* 6, 3 (2015): 87–97.

92 K. Uvnäs-Moberg, L. Handlin, and M. Petersson, "Self-soothing behaviors with particular reference to oxytocin release induced by non-noxious sensory stimulation," *Frontiers in Psychology* 5 (2014), doi: 10.3389/fpsyg.2014.01529.

93 Victoria P. Barrett, *An Evaluation of Exogenous Oxytocin in Contrast to Alternative Methods of Labor Induction in Uncomplicated Pregnancies*, Senior thesis defense, Colorado State University–Pueblo, April 18, 2017.

94 http://americanpregnancy.org/labor-and-birth/birth-plan

95 Cynthia M. Bulik, Ann Von Holle, Anna Maria Siega-Riz, Leila Torgersen, *et al.*, "Birth outcomes in women with eating disorders in the Norwegian Mother and Child Cohort Study (MoBa)," *International Journal of Eating Disorders* 42, 1 (2009): 9–18.

96 Veronica Bridget Ward and Deborah Waller, "Eating disorders in pregnancy," *British Medical Journal* 336, 7636 (2008): 93–96.

97 H. Lowes, J. Kopeika, N. Micali, and A. Ash, "Anorexia nervosa in pregnancy," *The Obstetrician & Gynaecologist* 14 (2012): 179–187.

98 Ibid.

99 Pam England and Rob Horowitz, *Birthing from Within: An Extra-Ordinary Guide to Childbirth Preparation* (Albuquerque, NM: Partera Press, 1998).

100 Fourth Trimester Podcast, "Listen to this if you are considering hiring a doula: What to expect with Monique the doula," February 11, 2018, www.fourthtrimesterpodcast.com/2018/02/listen-to-this-if-you-are-considering-hiring-a-doula-heres-a-day-in-the-life-of-monique-the-doula.html

101 Ibid.

102 Heng Ou, Amely Greeven, and Marisa Belger, *The First Forty Days: The Essential Art of Nourishing the New Mother* (New York, NY: Stewart, Tabori, and Chang, 2016).

103 Lourdes Alcañiz, "Bringing back the Hispanic tradition of 'cuarentena' after childbirth," Babycenter.com, www.babycenter.com/0_bringing-back-the-hispanic-tradition-of-cuarentena-after-chi_10346386.bc

Chapter 6

104 Tongue tie (ankyloglossia) is a medical condition some babies are born with. Babies with this condition may have trouble sucking, latching, gaining weight, and, later, speech problems. Tongue clipping is a surgery to treat tongue tie.

105 Kathryn Dewey and Caroline Chantry, "Breastfeeding fraught with early challenges for most first-time mothers," UCDavis Health, September 23, 2013, http://ucdmc.ucdavis.edu/publish/news/newsroom/8223

106 Penny Simpkin and Phyllis Klaus, *When Survivors Give Birth: Understanding and Healing the Effects of Early Sexual Abuse on the Childbearing Woman* (Seattle, WA: Classic Day Publishing, 2005).

107 Caroline Bologna, "Mom seeks legal action after being 'humiliated' for breastfeeding on plane," *Huffpost*, February 5, 2016, www.huffingtonpost.co.uk/entry/mom-seeks-legal-action-after-being-humiliated-for-breastfeeding-on-plane_us_56b4d8cbe4b01d80b2460667

108 Anna Quindlen, "Public and private: To feed or not to feed," *New York Times*, May 25, 1994.

109 Katia Hetter, "Breastfeeding mom says flight traveled to unfriendly skies," *CNN Travel*, March 13, 2015, www.cnn.com/travel/article/feat-united-airlines-breastfeeding-incident/index.html

110 Ibid.

111 "Is it safe for mothers to use prescription medications while breastfeeding?" Centers for Disease Control and Prevention (CDC), www.cdc.gov/breastfeeding/breastfeeding-special-circumstances/vaccinations-medications-drugs/prescription-medication-use.html

112 Ibid.

113 Teri Pearlstein, Margaret Howard, Amy Salisbury, and Caron Zlotnick, "Postpartum depression," *American Journal of Obstetrics & Gynecology 200*, 4 (2009): 357–364.

114 Louann Brizendine, *The Female Brain* (Portland, OR: Broadway Books, 2006).

115 Michaleen Doucleff, "Considering breast-feeding? This guide can help," *NPR Shots*, June 27, 2017, www.npr.org/sections/health-shots/2017/06/27/534123212/considering-breast-feeding-here-s-how-to-make-it-easier

116 Michaleen Doucleff, "Secrets of breast-feeding from global moms in the know," *KQED Morning Edition*, June 26, 2017, www.npr.org/sections/goatsandsoda/2017/06/26/534021439/secrets-of-breast-feeding-from-global-moms-in-the-know

117 Melanie Klein Trust: www.melanie-klein-trust.org.uk

118 www.melanie-klein-trust.org.uk/paranoid-schizoid-position

119 C. Naumburg, "The gift of the good enough mother," Psych Central, February 10, 2018, https://blogs.psychcentral.com/mindful-parenting/2013/09/the-gift-of-the-good-enough-mother

120 Geneen Roth, *Women, Food, and God* (New York, NY: Scribner, 2016).

Chapter 7

121 Postpartum Support International (PSI), "Perinatal Mood and Anxiety Disorders Certificate Training," Fresno, CA, October 17–18, 2013, www.postpartum.net

122 Norwegian Institute of Public Health, "Pregnant women with bulimia have more anxiety and depression, study finds," *ScienceDaily*, September 18, 2008, www.sciencedaily.com/releases/2008/09/080917095356.htm

Walter H. Kaye, MD (Eating Disorders Center for Treatment and Research, University of California San Diego, Eatingdisorders.ucsd.edu), in his talk "Using neurobiology to understand traits and improve treatment," discussed how the following are traits common to someone who develops an eating disorder: persistence, perfectionism, interoceptive awareness, obsessive personality, drive to thinness, negative emotion. International Association of Eating Disorder Professionals (iaedp) Symposium, St. Petersburg, Florida, February 27–March 2, 2014.

123 https://behavioraltech.org/about-us/founded-by-marsha
124 Elisha Goldstein, "Radical acceptance: An interview with Tara Brach," PsychCentral, September 2009, https://blogs.psychcentral.com/mindfulness/2009/09/radical-acceptance-an-interview-with-tara-brach
125 Ibid.
126 www.dbtselfhelp.com/html/overview1.html
127 Bessel van der Kolk, *The Body Keeps the Score: Trauma Healing*, PESI workshop, San Francisco. CA, April 2017.

Chapter 8
128 Stephanie S. Covington, *A Woman's Way through the Twelve Steps* (Center City, MN: Hazelden, 1994).
129 Ibid.
130 Andrea Wachter and Marsea Marcus, *The Don't Diet, Live-It Workbook: Healing Food, Weight and Body Issues* (Carlsbad, CA: Gürze Books, 2010).
131 Gürze interview with Carolyn Costin and Joe Kelly, "Yoga and Eating Disorders: Ancient Healing for Modern Illness Interview," October 31, 2016, www.edcatalogue.com/yoga-eating-disorders-ancient-healing-modern-illness-interview
132 Denise Roy, *Momfulness: Mothering with Mindfulness, Compassion, and Grace* (San Francisco, CA: John Wiley and Sons, 2007).
133 http://juliacameronlive.com/basic-tools/morning-pages
134 www.dbtselfhelp.com/html/radical_acceptance_part_1.html
135 Jon Kabat-Zinn and Myla Kabat-Zinn, *Everyday Blessings: The Inner Work of Mindful Parenting* (New York, NY: Hachette Books, 2014).
136 http://self-compassion.org/the-three-elements-of-self-compassion-2
137 You can find Jennifer at ChimeYogaTherapy.com
138 www.handinhandparenting.org/tag/special-time
139 https://jackkornfield.com/meditation-lovingkindness
140 Jack Kornfield, *The Art of Forgiveness, Lovingkindness, and Peace* (New York, NY: Bantam, 2002).
141 Denise Roy, *Momfulness: Mothering with Mindfulness, Compassion, and Grace* (San Francisco, CA: John Wiley and Sons, 2007).
142 Ibid.
143 Jon Kabat-Zinn and Myla Kabat-Zinn, *Everyday Blessings: The Inner Work of Mindful Parenting* (New York, NY: Hachette Books, 2014).

Chapter 9

144 Leslie Morgan Steiner, *Mommy Wars: Stay-at-Home and Career Moms Face Off on Their Choices, Their Lives, Their Families* (New York, NY: Random House, 2007).

145 Samantha Parent Walravens, *Torn: True Stories of Kids, Careers, and the Conflict of Modern Motherhood* (Seattle, WA: Coffeetown Press, 2011).

146 In the 1960s, Harry Frederick Harlow, an American psychologist, performed (ethically questionable) experiments on infant rhesus monkeys, testing maternal separation, dependency, and social isolation effects. In one experiment, a "wire mother" monkey held a bottle with food, and a "cloth mother" held no food. The infants chose to stay with the cloth mother for comfort, leaving her only when food was required.

147 Melissa Arca, MD, FAAP, "Working mom: The highs and lows as captured by a 6-year-old," Confessions of a Dr. Mom, January 22, 2014, www.confessionsofadrmom.com/2014/01/working-mom-the-highs-and-lows-as-captured-by-a-6-year-old

148 Rachel G. Lucas-Thompson, Wendy A. Goldberg, and JoAnn Prause, "Maternal work early in the lives of children and its distal associations with achievement and behavior problems: A meta-analysis," *Psychological Bulletin* 136, 6 (2010): 915–942.

149 Caitlin Moscatello, "Cloudy…with a chance of rage?" *Oprah Magazine*, February 2014.

150 self-compassion.org; Kristin Neff, *Self-Compassion: The Proven Power of Being Kind to Yourself* (New York, NY: HarperCollins, 2011).

151 Donna Reed was an American movie and television actress who played the "perfect" mother and wife on *The Donna Reed Show* in the 1950s and 1960s.

152 Lonnae O'Neal Parker, "The Donna Reed Syndrome: High pressure, demanding bosses, cutthroat politics – boy, it's hard work staying at home," *Washington Post*, May 12, 2002.

153 Arlie Hochschild and Anne Machung, *The Second Shift* (New York: Penguin, 2003).

154 Claire Cain Miller, "Women at Work: Mounting evidence of advantages for children of working mothers," *New York Times*, May 15, 2015.

155 Lydia Denworth, "Fluidity," in Samantha Parent Walravens (ed.) *Torn: True Stories of Kids, Career and the Conflict of Modern Motherhood* (Seattle, WA: *Coffeehouse Press*, 2011), http://lydiadenworth.com/books/torn/fluidity

156 Ibid.

Chapter 10

157 M. Mills, R.R. Rindfuss, P. McDonald, P.E. te Velde, ESHRE Reproduction and Society Task Force, "Why do people postpone parenthood? Reasons and social policy incentives," *Human Reproduction Update* 17, 6 (2011): 848–860.

158 Rebecca Dekker, Mimi Niles, and Alicia A. Breakey, "Evidence on: Advanced Maternal Age," Evidence Based Birth®, March 29, 2016, https://evidencebasedbirth. com/advanced-maternal-age

159 Ibid.

160 B. Mangweth-Matzek, H.W. Hoek, C.I. Rupp, K. Lackner-Seifert, et al., "Prevalence of eating disorders in middle-aged women," International Journal of Eating Disorders 47, 3 (2014): 320–324.

161 Adriana Barton, "Are middle-aged women succumbing to 'Desperate Housewives syndrome'?" The Globe and Mail, May 1, 2011, updated May 11, 2018, www.theglobeandmail.com/life/health-and-fitness/are-middle-aged-women-succumbing-to-desperate-housewives-syndrome/article578178

162 Glenn E. Palomaki, Edward M. Kloza, Geralyn M. Lambert-Messerlian, James E. Haddow, et al., "DNA sequencing of maternal plasma to detect Down's syndrome: An international clinical validation study," Genetics in Medicine 13 (2011): 913–920.

163 Anne-Marie Nybo Andersen, Jan Wohlfahrt, Peter Christens, Jørn Olsen, and Mads Melbye, "Maternal age and fetal loss: Population based register linkage study," British Medical Journal 320, 7251 (2000): 1708–1712.

164 Ling Huang, Reg Sauve, Nicholas Birkett, Dean Fergusson, and Carl van Walraven, "Maternal age and risk of stillbirth: A systematic review," Canadian Medical Association Journal 178, 2 (2008): 165–172.

165 M. Jolly, N. Sebire, J. Harris, S. Robinson, and L. Regan, "The risks associated with pregnancy in women aged 35 years or older," Human Reproduction 11 (2000): 2433–2437.

166 Tracey A. Mills and Tina Lavender, "Advanced maternal age," Obstetrics, Gynaecology & Reproductive Medicine 21 (2011), 107–111.

167 Jessica E. Tearne, "Older maternal age and child behavioral and cognitive outcomes: A review of the literature," Fertility and Sterility 103, 6 (2015): 1381–1391.

168 Shelly Grabe, Clay Routlege, Alison Cook, Christie Andersen, et al., "In defense of the body: The effect of mortality salience on female body objectification," Psychology of Women Quarterly 29, 1 (2005): 33–37.

169 Ann Harding, "Eating disorders: Not just for the young," Health.com, June 27, 2012, www.cnn.com/2012/06/26/health/mental-health/eating-disorders-not-just-for-young

170 Sheira Kahn and Nicole Laby, Erasing ED Treatment Manual: Tools and Foundations for Eating Disorder Recovery (North Charleston, SC: CeateSpace, 2012).

Index